THE
BLACK
DEATH
IN LONDON

THE
BLACK
DEATH
IN LONDON

BARNEY SLOANE

The
History
Press

'In the year of Our Lord 1349, a violent pestilence broke out beyond measure in the whole of the Kingdom of England, and especially in the City of London, where the people superabounded. So great a multitude eventually died that all the cemeteries of the aforesaid city were insufficient for the burial of the dead. For this reason, many were compelled to bury their dead in places unseemly, not hallowed or blessed; some, it was said, cast the corpses into the river.'[1]

Cover illustration: An engraving from *An Introduction to English Church Architecture from the Eleventh to the Sixteenth Century* (Volume 2) by Francis Bond.

First published 2011

The History Press
The Mill, Brimscombe Port
Stroud, Gloucestershire, GL5 2QG
www.thehistorypress.co.uk

British Library Cataloguing in Publication Data.
A catalogue record for this book is available from the British Library.

ISBN 978 0 7524 2829 1

Typesetting and origination by The History Press
Printed in the EU for The History Press.

CONTENTS

FOREWORD

THE FIRST onslaught of the Black Death in 1347–53 remains the greatest single catastrophe to have struck mankind in recorded history. A vast literature exists which examines and often vigorously debates its origins, its causes and its impacts on cities and manors, on economies and society, and on the very beliefs held by people over 600 years ago. Internationally, two major recent studies, Ole Benedictow's *The Black Death 1347–53: A Complete History* and Sam Cohn's *The Black Death Transformed*, set both the European stage and readily demonstrate the vigour of the debate.[2] England itself has been particularly well served since Francis Gasquet's treatise as long ago as 1893 on *The Great Pestilence*, and more recently by Philip Ziegler's highly readable *The Black Death* (1969), the essays in Mark Ormrod and Philip Lindley's *The Black Death in England*, and Colin Platt's *King Death* (both 1996); as well as a host of more detailed articles. London, however, is less visible in detail, although both Jens Röhrkasten and Barbara Megson have made important contributions to the study of the city's mortality during plague outbreaks.[3]

As a professional archaeologist, I came face to face with the effects of the epidemic on London during excavations at the Black Death cemetery of East Smithfield near the Tower of London, which unearthed hundreds of skeletons of the victims. But remarkably, given the relative abundance of its documentary records, the detailed story of how London succumbed, suffered and eventually adapted to this awful disease has never been told. This attempt to fill that gap reveals some rather surprising aspects of the city's reaction to the plague, it raises some fundamental questions about the level of mortality and it examines the later outbreaks (1361, 1368 and 1375) that dogged the reign of Edward III to set out comparisons and contrasts with the first terrible blow.

This book is not specifically about the causes of the plague, its identification with one or another pathogen, or the science of its spread (although a summary of current debate is provided). Rather, it has been my aim to develop a detailed historical narrative from documents and archaeology to provide as complete an understanding of the horrifying test to which the nation's capital was put. I hope that this analysis provides a springboard for further research into the impact of the Black Death on London. This is an essentially human story populated with many names of real people who came face to face with one of our worst nightmares and lived, or died, in London more than six centuries ago.

Barney Sloane

ACKNOWLEDGEMENTS

I WISH to thank specific organisations, friends and colleagues who have helped me considerably in the development of this book. First and foremost I would like to acknowledge a debt of gratitude to Caroline Barron (Royal Holloway) who provided encouragement and many very helpful suggestions in developing the text. Christopher Phillpotts reviewed and transcribed the relevant surviving manorial documents for Stepney. Claire Martin and Jeremy Ashbee gave their valuable time to undertake further examination and transcription of original documents. For further contributions to the historical research, I would like to thank Dr Mark Forrest for sharing his data on Gillingham in advance of publication. Ann Causton, Robert Braid, Sam Cohn, Graham Dawson and Penny Tucker provided further help. I have benefited greatly from the generosity of archaeologists involved in the excavation or analysis of material from this period, and here I would very much like to thank Ian Grainger and Chris Thomas of the Museum of London Archaeology, the late Bill White of the Centre for Human Bioarchaeology at the Museum of London, and Dr Sharon DeWitte (Albany University). For additional advice in structuring the text and contents I record my gratitude to Professor Roberta Gilchrist (University of Reading), and Dr John Clark (Museum of London); and for helpful comments I would like to thank Jenni Butterworth, Nathalie Cohen, Peter Mills, and Professor James Wood. I am very grateful for use of photographs and graphics prepared and/or supplied by Carlos Lemos and Andy Chopping (Museum of London Archaeology), and Dr Jeremy Ashbee.

ABBREVIATIONS

Arch J	Archaeological Journal
CAD	H.C.M. Lyte (ed.), 1915, *A Descriptive Catalogue of Ancient Deeds*, Vol. 6 (London)
CAN	H. Chew & W. Kellaway (eds), 1973, *London assize of nuisance 1301–1431: A calendar*
CCR	*Calendar of Close Rolls*
CCRBL	W.H. Turner, 1878, *Calendar of Charters and Rolls preserved in the Bodleian Library* (Oxford)
CCRC	R.R. Sharpe (ed.), 1913, *Calendar of the Coroners' Rolls of the City of London AD 1300–1378* (London)
CFR	Anon, 1921, *Calendar of the Fine Rolls preserved in the Public Record Office, Volume VI, Edward III, 1347–56* (London)
CHW	R.R. Sharpe (ed.), 1889, 1890, *Calendar of wills proved and enrolled in the Court of Husting 1258–1688*, 2 Vols (London)
CIPM	H.C.M Lyte (ed.), 1916, *Calendar of Inquisitions Post Mortem, Vol. IX, Edward III* (London)
CLB F	R.R. Sharpe (ed.), 1904, *Calendar of Letter-books preserved among the archives of the corporation of the City of London: Letter-book F c. AD 1337–1352* (London)

CLB G	R.R. Sharpe (ed.), 1905, *Calendar of Letter-books preserved among the archives of the corporation of the City of London: Letter-book G c. AD 1352–1374* (London)
CLB K	R.R. Sharpe (ed.), 1911, *Calendar of Letter-books preserved among the archives of the corporation of the City of London: Letter-book K Temp Henry VI* (London)
CLPA	H. Chew (ed.), 1965, *London Possessory Assizes: a calendar* (London Rec Soc Vol. I)
CPL	W.H. Bliss & C. Johnson, 1897, *Calendar of entries in the Papal Registers relating to Great Britain and Ireland: Papal Letters, Vol. 3, AD 1342–1362* (London)
CPMR	A.H. Thomas (ed.), 1926, *Calendar of the Plea and Memoranda Rolls of the City of London, Vol. I, 1323–1364*
CPP	Calendar of Papal Petitions
CPR	Calendar of Patent Rolls
Fasti	*Fasti Ecclesiae Anglicanae 1300–1541*: Vol. 5 (St Paul's, London, 1963)
Foedera	T. Rymer, 1741, *Foedera, conventiones, literae, et cujuscunque generis acta publica, inter reges Angliae et alios quosvis imperatores, reges, pontifices, principes, vel communitates, ab ineunte saeculo duodecimo, viz. ab anno 1101. ad nostra usque tempora, habita aut tractata: ex autographis, infra secretiores Archivorum regiorum thesaurarias per multa saecula reconditis, fideliter exscripta*, Vol. 5
Hist Gaz	D.J. Keene & V. Harding, 1987, *Historical gazetteer of London before the Great Fire: Cheapside; parishes of All Hallows Honey Lane, St Martin Pomary, St Mary le Bow, St Mary Colechurch and St Pancras Soper Lane* (London)
LMA	London Metropolitan Archive
MOSJ	Museum of the Order of St John, Clerkenwell, London
PLoS Pathog	Public Library of Science: Pathogens Journal (www.plospathogens.org/home.action)
Proc Archaeol Inst	Proceedings of the Archaeological Institute
PROME	C. Given-Wilson, P. Brand, A. Curry, R.E. Horrox, G. Martin, W.M. Ormrod, J.R.S. Phillips, 2005, *The Parliament Rolls of Medieval England, 1275–1504* Leicester, Scholarly Digital Editions (CD-ROM)

TLAMAS	Transactions of the London and Middlesex Archaeological Society
TNA	The National Archive
VCH London 1	W. Page (ed.), 1909, *A history of the county of London*: Vol. 1: London within the Bars, Westminster and Southwark
VCH Middx 1	W. Pugh (ed.), 1969, *A history of the county of Middlesex*, Vol. 1
VCH Middx 2	W. Page (ed.), 1911, *A history of the county of Middlesex*, Vol. 2
VCH Middx 5	T.F.T. Baker & R. Pugh (eds), 1976, *A history of the county of Middlesex*, Vol. 5
VCH Oxford 4	A. Crossley & C.R. Elrington (eds), 1979, *A history of the county of Oxford*, Vol. 4: The City of Oxford
WAM	Westminster Abbey Muniments
WSA	Wiltshire and Swindon Archives

INTRODUCTION

C HARACTERISING THE specific history of epidemics, whose
durations are measured in months, requires consideration of detail.
There is therefore only space for the briefest introduction to fourteenth-century London and its hinterland in this book, and the numerous
place names and subjects that are mentioned within it will lead some read-
ers to wish to know much more of the topography and functioning of the
city. I would recommend firstly Caroline Barron's excellent book on *London
in the Later Middle Ages*, which sets the social, economic and administrative
scene, and Chris Thomas' study of *The Archaeology of Medieval London* to provide a feel for the physical nature of the fourteenth-century city. To this
I would add the very useful *British Atlas of Historic Towns: City of London from
Prehistoric Times to c. 1520*, edited by Mary Lobel, with its unsurpassed maps
reconstructing the medieval layout of the city. Finally, the flavour of city life
evoked by Barbara Hanawalt's *Growing up in Medieval London: the Experience
of Childhood in History* provides a clear sense of daily life in the city. There
is, of course, a formidable bibliography for medieval London, but just these
four will help bring a long-vanished city to life.

The historical evidence considered in this book has been drawn as far
as possible from detailed summaries of primary sources which have been
published in calendar form, augmented by some examination of the
original documents themselves. In accessing the calendars, I have made
much use of the superb British History Online initiative developed
by the Institute of Historical Research at University College London

(www.british-history.ac.uk), which provides full access to the calendars of the City of London Letter Books, the Pleas and Memoranda rolls of the mayoral court, the Possessory Assizes, the Assize of Nuisance and many other sources. I have also used the University of Iowa's online searchable edition of the Calendars of Patent Rolls (www.uiowa.edu/~acadtech/patentrolls), Tanner-Ritchie's searchable CD-ROM versions of the Calendar of Papal Letters, and the digital edition of the Parliamentary Rolls of Medieval England. In converting medieval feast days to modern equivalents (all dates have been rendered in the Gregorian system), I have made much use of the online regnal calendar for Edward III at www.medievalgenealogy.org. uk/cal/reg11.htm. One secondary source deserving of special mention, itself a collation of excerpts from primary medieval documents, is Rosemary Horrox's invaluable *The Black Death*.

The most important source for this study has been the two-volume Calendar of Wills Enrolled in the Court of Husting.[4] Covering the period 1259–1688, the wills are especially useful for the first three-quarters of the fourteenth century, and give us a superb insight into the arrangements made by the wealthier segment of the citizenry during the plague years.[5] What makes them particularly useful is the adoption, at the outset of Edward III's reign, of the practice of recording the date on which the will was actually drawn up. This information provides us with an effective means of gauging the level of threat that people considered themselves to be under, as well as the threat that they actually did face, and is therefore a unique barometer of the impact on London citizens at the time. Previous systematic studies of the evidence from this source have been aimed primarily at examining numerical trends, and most have not factored in the dates the wills were drawn up.[6] This considerably enhances our understanding of mortality trends during the outbreaks, as well as providing the intimate evidence, contained in hundreds of wills written or enrolled during the four outbreaks of pestilence between 1348 and 1375, of citizens as they prepared for and succumbed to the devastating disease. As with all historical documents, they have their limitations, and it is important to understand how the wills originated and how the court that enrolled them actually operated.

Wills were usually drawn up at a time when death seemed likely to the individual concerned. The priest who attended the dying to administer the last rites often also scribed the document. The will would then be kept by the individual or a nominated representative, to be presented by the executor or relative to the appropriate ecclesiastical court after death. The oversight of probate was reserved generally for the ecclesiastical courts, but at an early stage (and at least by 1258) the Husting court took charge of those wills which involved real estate within London owned and bequeathed by citizens.[7] Very few of the wills may have been enrolled during the lifetime of their makers – which would make their use in establishing death rates nonsensical – but we can be confident that this is a tiny fraction. The rolls into which these portions of wills were entered were used principally as proof of title to land and rents.[8] As such, they reflected the legal property interests of the wealthier London citizens and their heirs and executors.

The numbers of wills being drawn up and enrolled in Husting form an indicator of the general expectations, and experience, of mortality among the reasonably well-off and, by extension, may form a benchmark for the city as a whole. The percentage of Londoners that used the Husting court is very difficult to calculate. Between 1327 and 1348, the drawing up of wills and enrolments had each averaged around twenty-eight per annum.[9] If London's population in 1348 was 60,000 in all,[10] of which around 40 per cent were children and adult mortality was about 35 per 1,000 per annum (a figure estimated as reasonable for a pre-industrial society), then an average of 1,260 adults might be expected to have died each year. Of the annual average twenty-eight pre-plague Husting wills, they were predominantly (approx. 86 per cent) made by men.[11] So twenty-four male wills might be taken to represent 630 adult male deaths – almost 4 per cent. Of course, the picture is vastly more complex than this, as many who had been formally admitted as citizens did not actually live within the walls, but it is quite clear that the percentage is low. Nonetheless, for the fourteenth century at least, the Husting rolls provide a unique measure of the impact of successive plagues.

They also provide other valuable insights. Wills which came before the Husting had already been before one of the ecclesiastical courts to determine probate, so some delay might be anticipated between death and enrolment. This potential delay is significant. There is clear evidence (presented in the main text) for wills enrolled weeks, months, or possibly even years after their makers' deaths. Professor James Wood's examination of the time-lag apparent in filling vacant clerical benefices across England demonstrates clearly that the speed of the spread of the plague has been consistently and significantly underestimated;[12] sadly, the bishops' registers are missing for the whole diocese of London for the years 1337–61,[13] and all we have to balance this is a partial picture from the presentations made by the king during vacancies in monasteries. However, the wills evidence strongly supports this view, and it is likely that the speed of the passage of plague presented in this book may if anything be too slow. Crucially, though, the date recorded for the writing of each will acts as a *terminus post quem*, so the profile has an accuracy not achievable through other forms of record.

I have used the information in the Husting wills to assess wider changes in charity and religious belief, but to put this in context, it is important to understand that the nature of these wills was dynamic, and that considerable changes have been identified as dating to the periods 1339–50 and 1350 onwards. Before 1339 the wills were concerned primarily with immovable goods – essentially real estate. However, from about 1340, chattels and pecuniary bequests begin to feature much more commonly, and from 1350 onwards this trend is particularly marked. The reason for the shift is not clear but may have related to increased efforts to tax moveable goods.[14] This change means that assessing trends based on the comparison of pre- and post-pestilence wills requires caution.

For the two latest outbreaks of plague about which this book is concerned, those of 1368 and 1375, an increasing amount of information survives from the ecclesiastical courts. This includes the Archdeaconry Court wills (one incomplete register from 1368), dealing with London's 'middling sort', and with jurisdiction over about half of the parishes of the city (and a few nearby parishes such as Clerkenwell and Shoreditch); and the Commissary Court (beginning in 1373). The third ecclesiastical court relating to London, the Prerogative Court of Canterbury, contains wills only dated from 1383 onwards, so has not been used for this survey. Chance references in wills and charters indicate that spoken wills formed a notable part of Londoners' testamentary toolkit. These nuncupative wills clearly leave no primary documentary trace, but probates were entered in the registers of the ecclesiastical courts in the same manner as for written wills: between 1375 and 1400 the probates of over 380 such spoken wills are recorded.[15]

It is clear that the Husting wills, and indeed the other ecclesiastical registers, represent the response of the adult, propertied, and mainly male, segment of Londoners. We therefore translate the experiences in them across to the thousands of poor and the women and the children in the city and suburbs at considerable risk. Our sources for these, the majority of Londoners, are sadly limited. What survives includes a small number of intermittent, sometimes poorly preserved and unpublished court and account rolls from a handful of manors adjacent to the city. Many of these have not yet been examined but one, relating to the manor of Stepney,[16] provides important corroborative evidence which supports and amplifies that derived from the wills, and provides a remarkably coherent picture of the timing and impact of the disease.

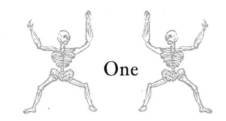

One

THE BEGINNING

OUTBREAKS OF disease were a fact of life in medieval London, and the term 'plague' or 'pestilence' covered a multitude of sins. One of the earliest medieval records of a Londoner dying of something called plague is that of the passing of Bishop Fulk Basset in 1259,[17] and epidemics in fourteenth-century London were, of course, known prior to the arrival of the Black Death.[18] They were occasionally of significant dimensions. The fifteenth-century *French Chronicle of London* recorded the 'great pestilence' among the survivors of the famine of 1315–16, while the chronicle of Henry Knighton, covering the years 1337–96, recorded how a plague in 1340 caused 'men to bark like dogs' with pain.[19] It was perhaps with this outbreak, or an undocumented more recent one, in mind that on Sunday 10 August 1343, it was proclaimed throughout the city that as part of measures introduced to keep the king's peace, 'All men of the misteries, as well as victuallers, journeymen, labourers and servants, shall work as they used to do before the pestilence, under pain of imprisonment and fine'.[20]

Whatever this pestilence was, it had clearly been sufficient to reduce the labour pool in the city, and the city's response to attempt to limit wages presaged the stringent statutory measures which would be introduced following the devastating pestilence of 1348–9. The early 1340s pestilence left no obvious trace within the wealthier will-making group represented by the Husting rolls;[21] it may of course have affected the poorer strata of the city more seriously than the wealthy, but it is noteworthy that a plague apparently significant enough to elicit a response from the city authorities regarding mortality levels could be otherwise invisible in the testamentary record. So the London of the 1340s had experienced epidemics, but that experience would not have prepared the citizens and residents for what was to come just a few years later. The years 1348 and 1349 were to witness the unfolding of the 'most lethal catastrophe in recorded history'.[22]

An Image of London in the 1340s

It is helpful to sketch out an image of London by way of setting the scene. The city in the reign of Edward III was by European standards impressive. By English standards it was a colossus, and it dominated national and overseas trade, political and courtly interests. In 1339, just a decade before the events described in this book, it was described as a 'mirror and example to the whole land'. A conurbation comprising the walled city, extensive suburbs, Southwark across the Thames, and Westminster, its resident population probably numbered near 80,000 souls in 1300, four times the size of Norwich, and ten times that of Great Yarmouth. It was the hub of an international trade network which brought merchants from across the known world by both land and sea. It boasted a very diverse economy, a complex civic administration that was emulated elsewhere, the largest concentration of religious houses, hospitals and friaries in the land, and crucially, at Westminster, the coalescing centre of national government.

Its walled circumference was essentially Roman, with the exception in the west of the westward bulge of the Dominican friary, and in the east the vastness of the Tower. At its spiritual heart lay St Paul's Cathedral, Romanesque at its core, but with considerable, newly completed work including one of the greatest spires in Europe dominating the skyline finished in 1314; nearby, a little to the north-east, stood the great Guildhall, seat of the principal civic administrative rulership in the form of the mayor and aldermen. The city's economic engine was the extensive waterfront, then a complex mixture of stone river walls and timber revetments, docks, wharves and cranes projecting outward into the highway that was the Thames. Vessels clustered around these, loading and off-loading the prodigious quantities of exports and imports, to be transferred away along bustling lanes such as Dowgate, Billingsgate and Oystergate up to the warehouses, shops and markets that lined the streets. Major markets could be found within the city, such as at the Shambles (meat market), Poultry (poultry market) and Cornhill (grain market); and major yearly fairs took place at, for example, West Smithfield (livestock) and Westminster Abbey.

The houses were a mixture of numerous fine stone mansions, such as John Poulteney's Coldharbour, or towered complexes such as Servat's tower at Bucklersbury, and the more modest wooden and stone tenements packing in perhaps 60,000 inhabitants in all in 1348. Gardens there were too, in numbers, with fruit trees and livestock regularly referred to in the documents, and some areas, especially the north-western quarter of the city, may have presented a surprisingly green aspect. Industry was everywhere, at a craft or cottage scale and sometimes on a more intensive basis as in Cripplegate in the north-west and St Mary Axe in the north-east, where archaeological evidence for metalworking covering multiple plots has been found.

One hundred and twenty parish churches served the religious needs of this teeming population with their belfries, fonts and churchyards for the dead, but as well as these, London's great influence had drawn the religious orders to found numerous monasteries and nunneries. Outside Aldersgate lay St Bartholomew's priory and hospital, and across the great livestock market at West Smithfield stood the great priory of St John of Jerusalem, the headquarters of the Knights Hospitaller, and the nunnery at Clerkenwell; west, towards Westminster, was the Carmelite (White) friary, and next to it, the halls and church of the disbanded Knights Templar, now filling with London's growing cadre of lawyers and appellants.

Inside Newgate stood the Franciscan (Grey) friary, not far from the Dominican (Black) friars against the extended city wall to the south, and even closer to the venerable college of St Martin-le-Grand. On the eastern side of the city gathered a similarly impressive group of monastic houses. St Helen's nunnery in Bishopsgate stood south of St Mary Bethlehem (of Bedlam fame), which in turn was neighbours almost with the great hospital priory of St Mary Spital, just beyond the gate itself. At Aldgate stood the impressive church and priory of Holy Trinity, and south and east of this stood, inside the walls, the house of the friars of the Holy Cross (the 'Crutched Friars'). Beyond them was the house of the sisters known as the Poor Clares, or Minoresses, Franciscan nuns who passed their name to the area of the Minories. Concluding the circuit, to the south-east of the Tower lay the third of the city's hospitals, that of St Katherine. Most of these were well established, having been founded as much as two centuries earlier, but two were very recent. The hospital and priory of St Mary founded by William Elsyng, the remains of whose church still stand on London Wall just east of the Barbican Centre, was less than twenty years old, and the college founded by Sir John de Pulteney, or Pountney, adjacent to the parish church that still bears his name, St Lawrence Pountney, was down towards the river.

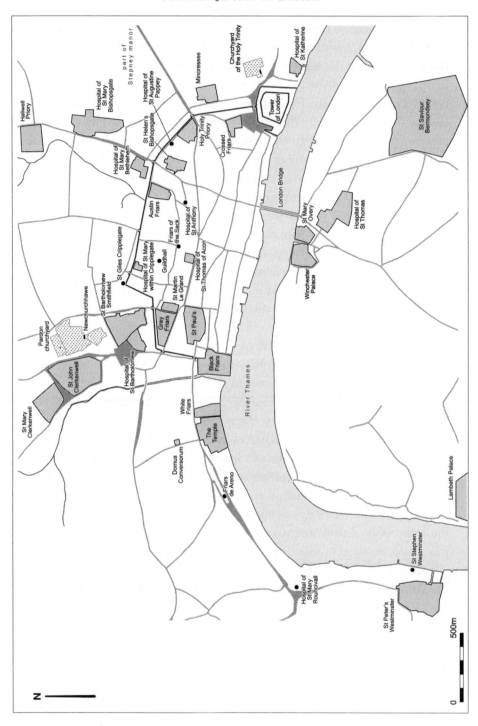

Fig. 1 A map of medieval London, including Westminster and Southwark, showing notable buildings and precincts and the emergency pestilence cemeteries of West and East Smithfield.

The prisons at this date, especially the Fleet prison and nearby Newgate, were fearsome places where, without external support, one ran the real risk of starving to death or being consumed by sickness. Equally feared was the humiliation, agony and significant risk of long-term damage from a few hours on Cheapside's famous pillory, with the rotting meat or counterfeit clothing burned beneath the villain's face: some would risk a prison sentence to avoid this particular punishment. The theft of two oxen and three cows from outside Aldersgate earned Thomas de Braye a hanging in March 1348, and the spikes of London Bridge held traitors' heads fresh from Tower Hill or Tyburn, or the less well-known execution site at Nomannesland out towards Clerkenwell.

From among the riverside quays the many-arched twelfth-century stone bridge spanned the Thames south to Southwark. This was considered a suburb by many, but with a population of perhaps 5,000 it was large enough to justify being called a town.[23] The houses, including some fine mansions such as that of the Prior of Lewes, clustered near the bridgehead and along the main north–south road, or, like Dunley's Place, along the waterfront.[24] The settlement had several parish churches and two important religious houses – the Cluniac monastery at Bermondsey to the east and, near the bridgehead, the Augustinian priory of St Mary Overy. To the west of the priory lay the extensive waterfront palace of the Bishop of Winchester. The hospital of St Thomas lay set back from the main high street, and at the extreme southern end of the settlement could be found the leper hospital known as The Lock. Southwark was the site of numerous brothels, and by the 1370s held two prisons – the King's Bench and the Marshalsea.

Westward from the city extended a ribbon development along Fleet Street and the Strand towards Westminster. By the fourteenth century this road was lined with the mansions of the elite, of earls, dukes and bishops such as those of Carlisle, Norwich and Durham, linking the economic powerhouse of the city with the centre of national government now firmly established at Westminster Palace.[25] Among these houses, closer to the city, stood the great Temple, the former house of the dissolved Knights Templar, and in the mid-fourteenth century leased out by the subsequent owners, the Knights Hospitaller, to lawyers and appellants serving the city and the court. Suitably isolated to the north of this thoroughfare was the leper hospital of St Giles-in-the-Fields, near the junction of modern Charing Cross Road and New Oxford Street.

Westminster itself was dominated by the royal palace and the great abbey, forming the heart of government in the kingdom. It is easy to forget that the town was significant in its own right with a population probably exceeding 3,000 before the plague.[26] It too had a parish church, a leper hospital at

St James in the Fields, and a hospital for the sick at St Mary Rounceval, near Charing Cross.

These three principal hubs of urbanism were, of course, ringed by numerous manors, with their attendant villages and hamlets, such as Islington, Tottenham, Stepney, Kingsbury and many more, sited on or near the main highways that brought the trade of the nation into the heart of London. The manor houses were often owned by London citizens, forming rural retreats away from the hubbub of city life.

This was London on the eve of the pestilence.

The Threat to England

The Black Death had already begun its spread across Europe as early as 1347, and its march has been charted elsewhere.[27] Its route to Britain was almost certainly from France, and we know that by January 1348 it had started killing people in Avignon. Toulouse and Perpignan were affected by April, Lyons in May, Givry in July, and Bordeaux and Paris by August. Seaborne infection had seen deaths beginning in Rouen in late June, although Caen does not appear to have been affected until September, and Calais not until December.[28] This rate, though terrifyingly rapid for those caught up in it, did provide sufficient time for the knowledge to spread and for the implications to be considered at the highest levels. Many Londoners must have known of the impending threat weeks or even months before it arrived. England was a trading nation and one at war with its neighbour; despite the obvious interruptions to cross-Channel communications that accompanied the conflict, many merchants in the capital must have been aware that by spring 1348, city after French city was falling before the scourge. Pilgrimages to European shrines were an important part of everyday medieval life, and travellers returning from St James de Compostella, Rome, and other key religious centres that had been affected early on must also have brought tales of woe and destruction. We have to assume that knowledge of its approach was thus reasonably widespread in the city long before the disease itself made landfall, threatening to spread panic and terror.

It is, in fact, rather hard to establish exactly how early the threat did register with Londoners. The documentary evidence for very early intelligence is slight and oblique. We have no London pilgrim's accounts, no mention in administrative documents from the city, and, so far, no references in surviving merchants' documents. The earliest evidence appears in papal correspondence in late spring 1348. On 15 May King Edward sent a team of papal diplomats to visit Pope Clement VI at Avignon to negotiate an extension of the existing truce in the war between England and France. The team comprised John Carlton, chancellor of Wells Cathedral, Thomas Fastolf, Archdeacon of Wells and a papal chaplain, and, significantly for London, John de Reppes, prior of the London Whitefriars and papal envoy since 1343.[29]

This advance party was clearly intended to negotiate a stop-gap in the war; they were given power only to discuss a maximum of one year's extension to the truce, pending the intended dispatch towards the end of September 1348 of the Earls of Lancaster and Arundel, and the Archbishop of Canterbury, with a view to a more binding arrangement. It is Carlton's signal to the Pope that his mission was limited which provides us with the first clear evidence that, in English diplomatic circles at least, the potency of the pestilence was recognised. Acting on information received from Carlton before 30 May, the Pope wrote to Philip of France to exhort him likewise to send envoys to Avignon, stating that the archbishop and the two earls were due to come from England to the papal court at Michaelmas (29 September) to give their consent to the prolongation of the truce, 'unless hindered by the epidemic'.[30]

Since Carlton was the source of the information, de Reppes and Fastolf must have known, and it is almost certain that such a plan had been discussed in advance with Edward. We may therefore safely conclude that the English king and at least one London prelate both knew as early as May 1348 that an epidemic had gripped France, and that Englishmen abroad were at risk. The king most likely knew much earlier than this, but proof is wanting.

There seems to have been no further indication of English activity or preparation for any such crisis in June. In Europe, however, stresses were reaching breaking point. On 5 July, in response to a growing popular suspicion of the source of the plague and resultant violence against them in Germany and other countries, Clement VI attempted to protect Jews by the reissue of the Bull 'Sicut Judeis'.[31] While it clearly did not directly affect England in any substantive way, it is likely that knowledge of the Bull would have made its way there quickly, providing another route along which knowledge of the pestilence might have flowed to London. By the end of the month, the king's concerns over the plague and its effect on his subjects overseas were growing. On 25 July, following the election of William de Kenyngton to the abbacy of St Augustine Canterbury, Edward, 'in view of the war with France then imminent, the dangers of the ways and the peril of death, by letters patent prohibited [William] from going' to Rome to confirm his elevation.[32] The reference is oblique, and plague is not specifically mentioned, but the reinforcement of three kinds of danger, including 'peril of death', is strongly suggestive of prior knowledge of the damage being wreaked by the disease which had, by this date, reached northern France.

Royal concern was mirrored by that of the senior clergy of the land. That the threat was being discussed openly in northern England is made clear in a letter dated 28 July from William Zouche, Archbishop of York, to his official in that city.[33] He wrote: 'There can be no one who does not know, since it is now public knowledge, how great a mortality, pestilence and infection of the air are now threatening various parts of the world, and especially England.' Identifying its cause as the sinfulness of the people, he laid out the earliest strategic defence plans against the plague:

> Therefore we command, and order you to let it be known with all possible haste, that devout processions are to be held every Wednesday and Friday in our cathedral church, in other collegiate and conventual churches, and in every parish church in our city and diocese … and that a special prayer be said in mass every day for allaying the plague and pestilence.

A release of forty days of penance was offered for those accepting the indulgence and entering into the processions. This sense of urgency from a northern prelate is striking, as is the sense that only a long-term round of mass prayer was likely to succeed. The warnings had been made public across the largest religious province in the kingdom. If York was making preparations of this nature, how much more concerned must London, far closer to the danger, have been at this time.

The warnings became more urgent. On 17 August 1348 Ralph of Shrewsbury, Bishop of Bath and Wells (no doubt well-informed by John Carlton), communicated to his own archdeacons the fact that a 'catastrophic pestilence' had arrived in 'a neighbouring kingdom', and urged that 'unless we pray devoutly and incessantly, a similar pestilence will stretch its poisonous branches into this realm and strike down and consume its inhabitants'.[34] His proposed strategy of prayer was similar to, and perhaps based upon, Zouche's with processions and stations to be held at least every Friday in all churches in the diocese. King Edward was almost certainly keenly aware of the concerns both of Zouche and Ralph of Shrewsbury. Before 23 August 1348 he is reported to have given serious consideration to the 'pestilences and wretched mortalities of men which have flared up in other regions', and to have sent letters to the Archbishop of Canterbury, John Stratford, requesting prayers to be said throughout the province of Canterbury.[35] Stratford, whose responsibility it was to have communicated this royal request through his bishops, died (though not, as far as we can tell, of any plague) on 24 August, and as a result the transmission of the orders was delayed until the following month.

There is good reason to suspect that the king's serious consideration also extended to his own spiritual preparations for impending disaster. The chapel of St Stephen the Protomartyr in Westminster Palace had been under substantial renovation for a number of years, but was as yet incomplete. However, on 6 August 1348 Edward confirmed the establishment of a college comprising a dean and twelve canons, granting them his 'great inn' in Lombard Street in the city at the same time.[36] The king cemented this arrangement on 20 August through a grant for life to a number of his senior servants. Thomas Crosse, clerk of the Great Wardrobe, received the deanery; John de Chesterfield and John de Maydenstone, clerks, received the first and second prebends; and John de Buckingham, a chamberlain, the third.[37] On its own, this may simply have represented an appropriate time to move ahead with the foundation of the college, but it is striking that on the very same day, Edward also recorded his intention to enhance considerably the small college of eight canons at Windsor Castle. He determined that:

> the glory of the Divine Name may be exalted by more extended worship [by the addition of] a warden and president of the same, fifteen … other canons, and twenty-four poor knights, to be maintained of the goods of the chapel, with other ministers, under the rule of the warden, willing that the canons and ministers shall celebrate divine offices there, according to an ordinance to be made, for him and his progenitors and successors, in part satisfaction of those of whom in the last judgement he will have to give account.[38]

These two foundations would certainly have provided the king with a considerable personal intercessory armament against the impending scourge.

Despite these early intimations and preparations, life in the city appears to have continued as normal. Major building works continued, at St Stephen's Westminster and also in the abbey itself, where renovation of both the east and south walks of the cloister were approaching completion, at least part of which were most likely to have been overseen by William Ramsey, the chief royal architect.[39] At the Tower of London, a new water-gate, the Cradle Tower, was being constructed to permit direct royal access from the river into the fortress. This tower had been started early in 1348, and building was to continue throughout the plague's visitation. Its name may have derived from the presence of a drawbridge lowered outward to provide a landing stage for the royal barge and then raised to seal the outer entrance to the water-gate. It remains one of London's few surviving medieval structures confidently datable to this specific period.[40]

Commercial land transactions were frequent, and particular documents provide engaging pictures of London life in the weeks before the pestilence struck. For example, on 4 September, the king licensed the mayor, aldermen and citizens to grant in fee to John de Gildesburgh, a wealthy fishmonger, a lane called 'Desebournelane' in the parish of St Mary Somerset near Queenhithe, for the purpose of building houses. The lane ran 215ft down to the Thames and was 7ft wide. The grant was conditional on Gildesburgh inserting a gutter 'to receive and carry off at all seasons of the year, rainy or not rainy, the water from all the highways there running down into the lane in their wonted manner and descending to the Thames'.[41]

Evidence is plentiful for the backdrop of imports and exports of an enormous range of goods into London's port and through its gates. Arrangements for the repayment of a loan from hugely wealthy merchants to the king (principally to finance the war with France) give some indication of the quantities of material passing through the port. On 25 September the king issued a writ 'to the collectors of the custom of wool, hides, and wool-fells on the port of London, with an order to pay Simon de Garton and Hugh de Kynardeseye or to their attorneys 20s out of every sack of wool and of every 300 wool-fells and 40s out of every last of hides taken out of that port, out of the realm' until they had recouped £7,500 on behalf of the king's merchant financiers, Walter de Chiriton, Thomas de Swanlond and Gilbert de Wendlyngburgh.[42]

Controls on exports to Europe are revealed by exceptions made: on 10 September Alan de Aylesham, a merchant of King's Lynn, was licensed to take twelve packs of worsted cloth to Flanders from the port of London, notwithstanding the late ordinance that cloth must be taken to Calais and not elsewhere.[43] Far more modest commercial deals are also reflected in the documents of the time, such as the debt acknowledged on 23 September by Thomas Reyner, citizen and taverner of London, to Hamo the Barber, citizen and cornmonger of London, of £7 8s, presumably for advance stock.[44] Crafts and trades guilds appear in the documentary record for August: the pewterers' guild ordinances were drawn up and presented to the mayor and aldermen, and admissions to the guild of leatherers recorded in the City Letter Books, for example.[45]

The Great Wardrobe, the mechanism for managing the royal assets and provisions, is glimpsed in September. Edward issued a writ of aid for one year, for Thomas de Tottebury, clerk of Queen Philippa's great wardrobe, to bring timber from her parks of Havering-atte-Bower (Essex), Bansted (Surrey) and

Isleworth (Middlesex), and stone from the quarry of Tollesworth (Surrey), and from all quarries in the county of Kent by the towns of Maidstone and Aylesford on the Medway. Workmen were to cart and prepare the stone, and 'to cause the same to be brought to her wardrobe in "La Rioll" London, at her charges'.[46] La Riole was a substantial property in the parish of Great St Thomas Apostle, to which such imports occurred roughly yearly, both before and after the principal plague months, suggesting business as usual.

The continuing conduct of the war against France naturally remained a subject of considerable interest to London traders. Many would have been heartened to hear the proclamation on 11 September, transmitted by the sheriffs to the citizens, that a truce had been concluded with France for a term of six weeks, from 13 September to 25 October. However, negotiations for peace were by no means complete, and on 25 September the king gave a commission to William, Bishop of Norwich, the Earl of Lancaster, Robert de Ufford, Earl of Suffolk, Sir Walter de Mauny, and John de Carleton, to treat formally for peace with France. A successful outcome could not be depended upon, so simultaneously Edward was augmenting his forces in case of failure: on 1 October he issued a writ to the sheriffs of London (and the mayors and bailiffs of seventeen other sea ports) to unload merchant ships and send them to join the fleet.[47]

The Tower of London had several roles at this time, including acting as a royal palace, a storehouse, the site of the royal mint and as a royal prison. Both the latter are glimpsed when, on 26 September, the king instructed John Darcy, constable of the Tower, to release one Nicholas de Luk (de Lucca), lately a serjeant of Percival de Portico, master of king's money in the Tower. De Luk had been imprisoned there for accounting anomalies identified by de Portico, but had protested that he was able to fully account for any inconsistencies. Lacking any counter-argument from de Portico, the king ordered de Luk's release.[48] Another notorious London prison makes an appearance at this time, when an order was sent from the king to sheriffs of London to release William Talentyre, clerk, from Newgate prison, pending a court hearing on a charge against him of writing a charter with the king's seal attached, 'ingeniously abstracted from certain of the king's letters patent' and then fastened to that charter.[49]

London citizens themselves and the minutiae of their lives also surface in the documentary records, most commonly through personal disputes and the wills they left. Disputes over property came before the court known as the Assize of Nuisance, held at the Guildhall. On 26 September two complaints were heard by the mayor and aldermen, both touchingly 'modern' and familiar. The first was a party wall dispute of sorts. Alan Gille and John de Hardyngham, wardens of London Bridge, alleged that Thomas Isoude, rector of St Margaret Friday Street, removed a rain gutter on the south side of the church to build a kitchen, and replaced the old gutter with two new gutters, one to receive the water from the church, and the other, leading into it, the water and waste from the kitchen. However, the water from both fell instead upon the tiles and party walls of the Bridge tenement adjoining the church, causing foundations, walls and timber to rot. The rector was given forty days to remedy the situation.[50]

The second case was a very early example of an ancient lights dispute. William Peverel, Queen Philippa's tailor, complained that Matilda (Maud) atte Vigne had built a cellar, blocking the light of the windows in his tenement in the parish of St Clement Candlewickstreet opening on to her land and garden, which he was intending to enlarge. Matilda replied that she had built on her own land, as she was entitled to do, and that there was no case against her. William maintained that the former owner of her plot, Gilbert de Colchester, had granted by deed to William's predecessor, in perpetuity, the light of the windows overlooking her tenement, with the right to enlarge them at will, and he produced a deed sealed with Gilbert's seal. Matilda denied that any such arrangement was ever granted by Gilbert and declared that the deed was not his. The case was referred to the next Husting of Common Pleas.[51] The outcome remains a mystery; the Assize was not to hear petitions again for eight months.

Death was ever-present in the crowded city, and many wealthier citizens with property interests were accustomed to drawing up wills for enrolment in the Court of Husting. The summer of 1348 in London was unremarkable in terms of will-making, with two wills drawn up in July, five in August and six in September.[52] The court was suspended at harvest time (August and September) and for major fairs, but eight wills were enrolled in July 1348, which was not an unusual number for the height of summer. Another potential indicator of concern over matters of mortality, requests from wealthy citizens for papal permission to choose one's confessor at the hour of death, reveals no especial change from levels in previous years: two married couples, Simon de Berkyng and his wife Lucy, and Thomas Leggy, then Mayor of London, and his wife Margaret, received indults of this sort in July and August respectively,[53] but that was the sum total up to September 1348. By this date wealthy Londoners were neither dying in excessive numbers nor, it would appear, expecting to. To the east, the picture was similar for the poor customary tenants working the land of the Bishop of London's manor at Stepney. The periodical court rolls are incomplete, but the court held on 30 October 1348, covering areas of Stepney, Hackney, Mile End, Stratford and Holywell Street, reports no deaths from the previous court (undated, but probably at least a month earlier), confirming instead three tenements held in the lord's hands (due to earlier deaths of tenants, one at least dating back to September 1347).[54]

These reflections of London urban life in the summer and autumn of 1348 are just snippets, but taken together they provide a flavour of daily life and death in the busiest city in the land. None of the documents mention anything at all about the plague, but in just a few weeks, by All Hallows' Eve, this familiar social environment was to face potential obliteration.

An English Pestilence

The various chronicles suggest a date for the arrival of the plague in England between late June and late September. We must assume that what they meant by 'arrival' was the first appearance of the symptoms and the evidence of an abnormal death rate. The actual date of landfall may have been some days or possibly weeks earlier, when the pathogen was still in its incubation stage and its first human carriers were infectious but not displaying any symptoms.[55] However, there are no certain independent manorial or royal accounts of pestilence anywhere in England before October 1348, and I suggest here that the plague made its first English manifestation in late September or early October, and not in August.[56] The royal family itself may have received one of the earliest blows.

Preparations for the marriage of Edward's daughter Joan to Pedro, infante of Castile, had been under way since as early as 1 January 1348, with establishments that any male heir would inherit the title of King of Castile.[57] En route to Spain, Joan and her entourage departed Portsmouth in early August, arriving some time before the 20th. She perished of the plague on 2 September. Edward was probably at Clarendon when the news arrived, but had returned to Westminster before he wrote to the Spanish royal family. His letter, dated 15 October, makes clear his inward desolation caused by the 'sting of this bitter grief', but illuminates a brave face on the tragedy as he accepted that he had a daughter in heaven who can 'gladly intercede for our offences before God himself'.[58]

Nor was this the sum of Edward's personal woes. On 5 September, at a lavish and fully regal funeral, Edward's 3-month-old son, William of Windsor, was laid to rest in Westminster Abbey. The infant's body had been brought from Brentford (perhaps having been borne there by boat from Windsor) to London accompanied by fifty paupers 'of the King's alms', carrying torches, for which they were paid 1s each, and laid out in state in the abbey church. Curiously, the accounting for the paupers' expenses only appears in the Michaelmas term of Edward's twenty-third year; in other words, after the cessation of the plague over one year later.[59]

Probably through the insistence of a king spurred on by such personal disaster, on 28 September 1348 Robert Hathbrand, the prior of Christchurch Canterbury, acting during the vacancy of the Archbishopric, sent to Ralph Stratford, Bishop of London, the orders from Edward III originally sent to the late Archbishop Stratford in August. The letter is known as Terribilis, from its opening word.[60] In it Hathbrand underlines the imminent disaster: 'it is now to be feared that the ... kingdom is to be oppressed by the pestilences and wretched mortalities ... which have flared up in other regions'. Such language indicates that to his knowledge the disease had not yet attacked England. By way of rationalising the coming plague, Hathbrand suggested that God used such devices to 'terrify and torment men and so drive out their sins', and exhorted the bishop to organise sermons at suitable times, and processions every Wednesday and Friday to help pacify God through prayer. Those citizens partaking were to be offered indulgences granting them a reduction of their time in Purgatory. The bishop was personally to ensure that these measures were set in place throughout the city and diocese of London, to communicate to his fellow bishops in the southern province, and to report back to the prior before 6 January 1349 to explain what actions had been taken. Ralph Stratford received these instructions by 5 October 1348, and communicated them to, among others, the Bishops of Exeter and Hereford. There, the message was to be spread to the people 'during procession and sermon in the cathedral',[61] and it is thus very likely that this was the mechanism for informing Londoners, too.

We can be sure that by early October, all of London was aware that death was threatening southern England, and that the city now lay in its path. Quite possibly, the first infected carriers had already entered the city, and the inexorable, invisible spread had begun.

Geoffrey le Baker (d. c. 1360), a clerk of Swinbrook, Oxfordshire, in an important chronicle detailing the period 1303–56, claimed that the pestilence entered London on 29 September 1348.[62] A later annal from Bermondsey Abbey in Southwark, covering the years 1042–1432, repeats this date, but may have been based on le Baker's work. However, this date seems rather too early, given the circumstantial evidence from other sources. The number of wills Londoners drew up (six in October) and the number of papal assents to choose confessors does not paint a picture of fear or panic, even if they might hint at an increasing concern.

Four citizens receiving indults to choose their own confessors were Thomas Cavendish, a draper on Cheapside, and Nicholas Ponge, a vintner near Bishopsgate, and two relatives, Matilda and Robert White, the latter a canon of St Paul's Cathedral. In terms of the numbers of wealthy will-making Londoners who were dying, only two wills were proved.[63] Covering parishes immediately to the north and east of the city, the court of the Bishop of London's manor of Stepney, held on 30 October 1348, records no deaths whatsoever, in stark contrast to its next session in early December and subsequent ones.[64] So it must be concluded that as yet, the pestilence had not physically manifested in the city, even if its psychological presence may have begun to make itself felt.

Further indirect support for a lack of any increased mortality can be derived from the analysis of 193 probates listed for May 1347 through to November 1348 in the register of Hamo de Hethe, Bishop of Rochester, a diocese which encompassed parishes as close to London as Greenwich. The last entered probates date to 3 November 1348, and a steady monthly average of about nine probates characterises the sample. By 23 December, however, with 'the plague now raging', anyone within the diocese was empowered by papal licence to hear confessions of the victims.[65]

During October 1348, the war with France, negotiations over prison-ers captured during the king's Scottish campaigns – especially the young King David II – and other domestic matters seem to have taken up more of Edward's energies than any preparation for the plague itself. Perhaps, having established the framework for a spiritual response, he felt able to set the responsibility on the shoulders of the bishops. Certainly his business relating to London reveals no specific evidence of disaster. He remained at Westminster throughout most of October (certainly from the 4th to the 24th), and on the 8th he issued a writ to the sheriffs of London for proc-lamation to be made 'for such men-at-arms, hoblers, archers, and others, as were willing to serve the King abroad, to be at Sandwich on Sunday before the Feast of Saints Simon and Jude (28th October) at the latest'.[66]

Two days later, Edward issued safe conduct until summer 1349 for Joan, wife of David II of Scotland, to come to the Tower of London to keep her husband company, following it up with similar safe conduct until December for Thomas, Bishop of Caithness, to treat for David's liberation from the Tower (an effort that was unsuccessful).[67] On 12 October protection was also offered to the prior of Bermondsey (a Cluniac house still dependent on its French province, so 'alien'), to whom the king had given custody of the priory during the war with France; royal protection extended to the priory and its community. Similar consideration was given to alms-gathering activities by hospitals in London, and he issued royal protection for two years to the master and brethren of the hospital of St Thomas the Martyr in Southwark.[68] Lastly, an investigation into the theft of £188 worth of jewels and other items from a turret in the Tower, sometime between their deposition in 1347 and 25 October 1348, led the king to issue a formal pardon to Bishop William Edington of Winchester, also the king's treasurer, and to Thomas Crosse and John de Buckingham (canons of Edward's new college at Westminster), whose responsibility it was to manage such royal assets.[69] These issues and correspondences, focusing on current events and royal responsibilities, do not seem to accord at all with the image of a city already wracked by death and disease.

The clearest indication that the killer had not yet begun its harvest was the letter written on 24 October by the Bishop of Winchester while in his chambers in the episcopal palace on the west side of Southwark. The palace was a very substantial Thames-side residence and guaranteed the bishop excellent access to the city and Westminster on the far side of the river. Edington's letter, written to the prior and chapter of St Swithin's Winchester and to all other clergy in his diocese, was a call to spiritual arms to protect Winchester and its people. Known as 'A voice in Rama' in reference to the Massacre of the Innocents,[70] the letter conjured up stark and fearful imagery. Of the villages, towns and cities consumed by the plague, it mourns that 'all joy within them ceases, all sweetness is dammed up, the sound of mirth silenced, and they become instead places of horror ...' It confirmed the dreadful news that 'this cruel plague has now begun a ... savage attack' on England's coastal areas.

Edington, echoing Zouche, Shrewsbury and others, commanded that the monks gather in their choir on Wednesdays and Sundays, and recite the seven penitential psalms and the fifteen psalms of degrees on their knees. On Fridays, the community was to process through the market place singing the same psalms, and also 'the great litany instituted by the fathers of the church for use against the pestilence'. For the people of his diocese, though, the time for defence had passed: the plague was in all likelihood already among them.

To what Edington's 'great litany' refers is not exactly clear. It is obvious that a special processional prayer against the plague had been constructed. It may have been based in some form on the *missa pro mortalitate evitanda*, the Mass for avoiding the plague, which had been compiled by Pope Clement VI in Avignon.[71] This Mass promised 260 days of indulgence to all who heard it and were truly contrite and confessed, and guaranteed that all who heard it on five consecutive days, kneeling with a candle in their hands, would not succumb to sudden death. Its efficacy had apparently been proved in Avignon and surrounding parts. Whatever the content of the litany was, the letter itself, written in London, must surely demonstrate that the plague was as yet unfelt in the capital.

As October drew to a close, changes to civic administration were in train. Thomas Leggy's term at the Guildhall as London's mayor came to an end, and he was replaced by John Lovekyn.[72] It was to be Lovekyn's term that encompassed almost exactly the duration of the plague. Meanwhile, the king had selected John de Offord, then Chancellor of England, dean of Lincoln, and prebend of St Paul's Cathedral, as his preferred candidate for the Archbishopric of Canterbury. The Pope favoured the decision (despite the fact that the chapter at Canterbury wished another London canon, Thomas Bradwardine, to take his place). De Offord's selection was inevitable given his powerful support; once confirmed, he would gain access to the great London archiepiscopal palace at Lambeth, but he would not be able to retain all the properties held through St Paul's Cathedral: in a letter of 24 October to John de Carleton (the canon of Wells who helped negotiate the truce with France), the Pope reserved to the latter the canonry and prebend of Tottenhale, which de Offord would have to resign on his elevation.[73] This moated site stood on the site of the modern junction between Euston Road and Tottenham Court Road, and thus in easy reach of the main western route to the city, but it has now long since vanished completely. In contrast, Lambeth Palace, directly across the Thames from Westminster, still stands remarkably complete.

In late October, in a chamber near the heart of the palace, Robert of Avesbury, the archbishop's commissory clerk, was no doubt hard at work. Avesbury was probably London's most credible eye-witness chronicler to the unfolding disaster that encompassed the city, and it is in his *de Gestis Mirabilibus Regis Edwardi Tertii* that we are provided with the date of All Saints' Day, 1 November 1348, as the beginning of the visible signs of pestilence in the city, as it took root and 'daily deprived many of life'.[74]

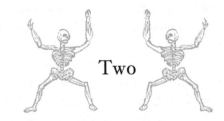

Two

THE PESTILENCE
IN LONDON

The City Infected, November 1348

THERE SEEMS little reason to doubt that Avesbury's date for the beginning of the nightmare was quite accurate. The making of wills suggests a significant increase at the very end of October: of the six wills drawn up in that month, four were dated to the last five days. Within three weeks, on 14 November, a papal indult was issued to all the clergy and people of both sexes of the city of London to permit them to choose confessors to give them plenary remission at the hour of death until Whitsuntide (31 May) 1349.[75] Such broad permissions as much as admit that the ability for the existing clergy to service the last rites of the populace would shortly be (or indeed already was) compromised beyond any capacity for regular management. It may, therefore, have been with some measure of relief to Edward that on 13 November his mission met with success in extending the French truce to 1 September 1349. The agreement was signed by the representatives of the two countries, including on England's side one Walter de Mauny, in Edward's tents just outside Calais.[76] Edward himself was not a signatory, but he was nearby and may have been present: in what has been described as a prominent propaganda exercise in the face of the oncoming pestilence, he had set sail for Calais on 29 October to see for himself what lay in store for his kingdom and his capital.[77] Having seen the appalling impact of the pestilence, he headed back from France for Sandwich on 17 November. The scale of the threat to his kingdom must now have been starkly clear and decisive action was needed.

On 20 November he issued a summons to Parliament to all the archbishops, twenty-one principal bishops, twenty-eight abbots of the larger monastic houses, and three priors, to discuss 'various urgent business (*urgentis negotiis*) and the state of our realm of England'. The summons to the Bishop of London warned that the dean and chapter of St Paul's, and the archdeacons and clergy of his diocese, should also be present; the dean and archdeacons in person, the others by proxy. On the same day, he issued orders for sheriffs in Cornwall, Somerset, Devon, Dorset, Southampton, Essex, London, Surrey, Sussex, Norfolk, Suffolk, Lincoln and Kent not to attempt to leave the country. These included the majority of southern and eastern coastal counties.

Three days later, on his return to Westminster, he issued orders effectively closing the ports of London, Dover, the warden of the Cinque Ports, Southampton, Newcastle, Harwich, Lynn, Ipswich, Rye, Boston, Shoreham, Great Yarmouth, Sandwich, Winchelsea and Kingston-upon-Hull; forbidding the crossing from England of any earl, baron, knight, squire or man-at-arms.[78] It is true that the news regarding France would have been of considerable import to those concerned with the management of the spiritual and temporal needs of the realm, and there would have been an urgent need to ensure no inadvertent truce-breaking by over-zealous commanders. However, the measures taken to ensure that peacekeepers and arms-bearers could not leave the country also point to a major internal issue. It seems highly likely that these commandments and convocations were focused as much on what the kingdom could do about the pestilence, and that the restriction of movement was intended to ensure that a solid command and control structure remained in place in the realm, and in particular at the great ports such as London, during the crisis.

If such were the king's plans, they were almost immediately confounded. The plague overwhelmed any intentions and, as will be seen shortly, the intended Parliament was never held. One man who might have expected to attend such a Parliament was Aleyn Ferthing, six-times Member of Parliament for the Borough of Southwark. His name is last mentioned in connection with a Parliament in 1348, and it seems certain that he perished in the epidemic. By chance, in 1832, workmen digging for a sewer on the site of the medieval church of St Margaret in Southwark found his Purbeck marble grave slab, inscribed *aleyn ferthing gist [ici dieu de son] alme eit merci amen*. It has been relaid in Southwark Cathedral,[79] and is probably therefore the only extant funerary monument in London made at the time of the plague.

The king was, of course, not alone in his preparations against the unseen killer now rampant in the kingdom. The number of Husting wills drawn up increased to ten in the month of November, and included several city worthies. Sir John de Pulteney, four times mayor and founder in the 1330s of the college of priests attached to the church of St Lawrence (afterwards called

Pountney), willed on 14 November the establishment of a chantry in St Paul's Cathedral, and made arrangements for the sale of his great mansion called 'Coldharbour' for a price of £1,000. John de Kelleseye, a goldsmith from the parish of St Mary Aldermary, by his will dated 11 November, instructed his wife to distribute every month for her lifetime seventeen silver pennies, one each to twelve poor men, three pence to a poor infirm man, and two pence to a poor woman. John de Hicchen, a pepperer and the rector of the church of St Antonin since at least 1345, willed on 28 November that a fraternity called the wardens of the Honour of St Anne should celebrate anniversaries for his soul, presumably in the chapel of St Anne in his church.[80]

Hicchen's will is particularly important. It was formally enrolled on 2 March 1349, but an addition on the will itself reveals that the actual date of his death was 2 December 1348, just four days after the will was drawn up, showing that enrolment could occur after a very considerable lag, and thus that many Londoners were very probably dying much earlier than the Husting enrolment evidence suggests. This lag explains why only three wills were enrolled in November, and none whatsoever in December. Indeed, it is only the dramatic rise in the number of wills made in December that indicate a catastrophe at all. The need for probate in the ecclesiastical courts prior to enrolment at Husting provides one reason for the lag, but it was almost certainly exacerbated by the plague itself: panic, death and confusion all would have led to changed priorities for survivors and a reduction in the operating efficiency of the courts. The significance of this lag relates clearly to our understanding of the actual speed of the plague's transmission within the city.

Another possible indicator of sudden death is a 'cluster' of three presentations of guardianship to the courts between late October and the beginning of December. The children of John Broun of Fleet Street were entered formally into the guardianship of his widow Elena on 23 October; Alice, widow of John de Lauvare, acknowledged the receipt of certain sums of money in trust for their children Robert, Simon and Richard on 14 November; and on 5 December Nicholas Bole, a skinner, acknowledged guardianship of the daughter of Simon de Pulham, whose widow Katherine he had married.[81] Wills do not survive for the three dead men, so we cannot be sure how recently they had perished, and furthermore such acknowledgements were not uncommon business in the courts. A cluster of three cases in seven weeks is, however, unusual.

The court of the Bishop of London's own manor of Stepney, lying immediately to the north-east of the city, convened on 9 December and provides clear evidence of rising mortality. Six deaths of customary tenants, all living in the parish of Hackney, had occurred since 30 October. They included three siblings of a single family, Sarra, Thomas and Richard Pymme, holding between them one cottage, a third of a toft and 3 rods of land. That they were poor is demonstrated by the fact that they had no animals to offer as heriot (a kind of death tax) to the bishop as their lord.[82] Bishop Edington took steps to save the souls of those who might die. On 17 November he wrote from his Southwark palace to his archdeacon in Winchester, granting to all rectors, vicars and chaplains across his diocese the right to hear confessions on account of the pestilence, requesting that they 'encourage recourse to the sacrament of penance on account of unexpected death'.[83] His diocese, of course, encompassed all of Surrey and thus numerous villages on the south bank of the Thames near London.

It is difficult to imagine what Londoners were facing during these first weeks of the plague. The disease and winter arrived in the city together, in a year already renowned for its storms and constant rain. John of Reading, a monk at Westminster during the plague (and another London eyewitness), wrote that rain had covered the south and west of England 'from Midsummer to Christmas, scarcely stopping by day or night'.[84] Short grim days and long dark nights set the scene for the unfolding horror. The knowledge that the plague was at hand would have sharpened a general fear into outright terror; every cough or twinge of pain a potential sign that a foul end was at hand. Reports would have spread through the city of the first deaths, perhaps down by the waterfront, or near the city gates; people may have tried to flee infected quarters or streets, before new deaths in previously untouched places set aside any thought of escape.

London's experiences cannot have been too much different from other European cities, so we can envisage household after household ripped apart by the appearance of the symptoms on husband, wife, mother, sibling or child. Realising that the contagion had settled on them, did each, as in Piacenza,[85] call out to friends and neighbours, 'Have pity, have pity, my friends … say something, now that the hand of God has touched me'? Did they reach out to relatives drawing away in fear of becoming infected themselves? Did they call for water, and plead not to be abandoned for dead; plead for someone to hold them tight and comfort their wracked bodies?

Few who contracted the disease would survive for long. The symptoms as described in Piacenza in early 1348 must have been truly terrifying to witness. First a chilly stiffness and tingling spread through the body, then, often, the buboes, up to the size of an apple, made their appearance in the armpit or the groin, growing, hardening and burning with a fiercely intense pain. Fever consumed the victim, accompanied by an intolerable stench. Vomiting or spitting of blood and further swellings or blotches of dark blood on the skin surfaces were followed by collapse and a final coma. Geoffrey le Baker noted of English victims that, rather than developing buboes, some 'had little black pustules scattered over the skin of the whole body', and observed that of these very few indeed survived.[86] The rapidity of the disease meant that the fate of the victim was decided in five days or less, most commonly three, a period confirmed by the Lambeth Palace clerk Robert of Avesbury, and another London eye-witness, Westminster monk John of Reading, who noted that 'ulcers broke out in the groin or armpit which tortured the dying for three days'. The disaster chiefly overwhelmed the young and the strong, according to le Baker, 'and hardly anyone dared to have anything to do with the sick'.[87]

In Florence a range of responses to the plague were observed in the citizens.[88] Some stockpiled food and water and closed themselves off in their homes, refusing to speak with anyone and hoping perhaps to wait out the onslaught. Some, unable to take in the enormity of what was happening, turned to drinking and carousing, often making use of deserted private homes as much as taverns. Other citizens tried to continue their lives as normally as possible, but equipped themselves with posies of flowers or herbs to ward off the evil humours of the disease. A final group abandoned everything and attempted to flee the disease by leaving the city. No doubt Londoners reacted in very similar ways but, just as in Florence, no matter what course they took, the awful harvest continued to grow.

There seems to have been no issue of any formal ordinances by the London authorities to attempt to stem or hinder the path of the plague, despite the strict instructions issued in several European towns earlier in the year. In Pistoia, strict ordinances were issued in the spring of 1348. No one was to travel to or from neighbouring towns such as Lucca or Pisa. No one was to transport or trade in used cloth of any sort. The bodies of the dead were to be placed in a wooden casket covered by a lid secured with nails, so that no stench could issue forth, before being moved; that casket was also to serve as the burial coffin. No one was to move the dead into or out of the city under any circumstances, and funerals were to be strictly limited in scale. Men from each quarter of the city were to be selected to move the dead – no one else was to undertake this; such men were to be paid out of city funds on production of a written receipt from the monastery, church or hospital to which the body was delivered for burial. The ordinances also set strict limits on butchery and tanning.[89]

At Tournai, in August 1349, city ordinances were issued, according to the Abbot of St Giles, as a result of the ineffectiveness of the secular clergy. They set out the following: concubines should either be married or put away under threat of banishment. The dead should be coffined and the grave dug immediately, regardless of the hour, but Masses should be saved up until Sundays; graves should be at least 6ft deep and the coffins not stacked up, and there should always be three graves ready per parish. Funeral feasts should be curtailed and gatherings at the house of the dead avoided. Finally, there were restrictions on trading after noon on Saturday until the following Monday.

By 21 September, further restrictions were imposed at Tournai, limiting the number of mourners to two per funeral.[90] Why London did not impose such constraints is not easy to establish, although it may relate to the more communal nature of civic government at this time. There is a level of archaeological evidence that wooden coffins were used more frequently for the burial of plague dead, suggesting that some guiding strategy may have been implemented (see Chapter 3).

Just one document hints at a public information system during plague outbreaks. A medieval parchment, found tucked into the wall of a rectory in Sherborne in the middle of the nineteenth century, provides a glimpse of the advice Londoners were given during the plague, communicated through a proclamation at the churchyard preaching cross at St Paul's Cathedral:

> Be it known to all Christian men and women that our Holy Father the Pope has true knowledge by revelation what medicine is for the sickness that reigneth now among the people. In any wise, when that you hear of this bull, first say in the worship of God, of Our Lady, and St Martin iii paternosters, iii aves, and i credo, and the morrow after immediately hear you the mass of St Martin and the mass while say ye the psalter of Our Lady and give one offering to St Martin, whatever that ye will, and promise to fast once a year in bread and water while you live, or else get another to do it for you. And he that believeth not of this stands in the sentence of Holy Church for it hath been preached at Paul's Cross.[91]

December 1348

The plague's impact on the city in December 1348 is quite clear from the twenty-seven Husting wills prepared during this one month (four written on a single day alone – 13 December). This represents a dramatic increase, nearly three times the rate of November and equivalent to an average year's total. This steep rise in mortality is also reflected in the one court roll for the year that we have from the suburbs – in this case the Bishop of London's manor at Stepney. In December 1348 four members of one family (mother, daughter and two sons) had died, and at the court held there on 20 January 1349, nine entire tenements were reported vacant and in the lord's hands owing to the death of the tenants.[92] To the south of the city, sudden clerical vacancies were filled by Bishop Edington at the churches of St Mary Magdalen, Southwark and Wandsworth in January, and in February at Clapham, Camberwell and St George the Martyr, Southwark, all less than 5 miles from Westminster. The Wandsworth institution recognised that, 'with the present increasing mortality, the bishop must provide for the needs of his flock'.[93] The deaths leaving these vacancies probably occurred in December and January, a conclusion strengthened by evidence from the court rolls for the manor of Vauxhall, a little more than half a mile from Lambeth Palace and probably held by Edward the Black Prince. The roll for the court held on 31 December 1348 recorded four deaths of customary tenants.[94]

Preferred burial locations and details of bequests set out in the wills indicate that the will-makers came from all different areas of the city, and from a wide range of professions. For example, Henry Iddesworth, canon of St Paul's and Archdeacon of Middlesex, made arrangements to leave his house in Wood Street and shops in the parish of St John Zachary towards the founding of a perpetual chantry in St Paul's Cathedral. Edmund de Hemenhale, a former sheriff of London and wealthy mercer, arranged for two executors to receive his estate in the 'great seld', or market, of Cheapside during the minority of John and Thomas, his sons, with a house in Lothbury set aside for John.[95] Edmund's family was still young: Thomas was 5 years old at this time, and a daughter, Margaret, was just 1.[96] Edmund was probably buried in St Martin-le-Grand, since his wife established there a chantry to them both when she died in 1361.

Geoffrey Penthogg, a waterbearer, willed on 30 December to be buried in the church of St Botolph Aldgate. He left his wife Johanna a messuage and a garden in the Portsoken ward, and his son John a garden in East Smithfield. He was dead within ten days, as Johanna's will, written on 9 January 1349, requested burial near her husband. Against this backdrop, and despite the (time-limited) blanket indulgence issued in November, some citizens continued to apply for papal permission to choose their confessors. Adam Pikeman and his wife Constance received permission in December, and Alexander de Bacland and his wife in January.

The wealthier were able to plan, afford and implement such arrangements for their goods and properties. They were able to choose the location of their graves, with at least some chance of getting their wishes even during the plague. This, however, did not apply to the vast majority of London's population. Being poor, they might normally expect a modest plot in one of the many small external cemeteries attached to parish churches in the city. But with mortality spiralling, it became clear to Ralph Stratford, the Bishop of London, that these, fairly numerous though they were, might not suffice for the disaster. Whether the concept of emergency cemeteries was due to have been discussed at the Parliament planned in November is unknown, but it is certain that between the outbreak of the plague in London and the end of December, Stratford had arranged for a new cemetery to be established on the city outskirts.

The chronicler Geoffrey le Baker described how the bishop bought the croft called by Londoners 'Nomanneslond'. This field lay south of another field called Whitewellbeck in the late thirteenth century, between modern St John Street and Goswell Road, and was apparently the site of executions from at least the early fourteenth century.[97] It measured some 3 acres, according to the sixteenth-century historian John Stow, and acquired the name of Pardon churchyard. It was apparently walled round and provided with a chapel.[98] This chapel is shown in remarkable detail on a sixteenth-century map of the water supply of the London Charterhouse; a three-bay, externally buttressed building with windows in each bay and a gabled roof surmounted by a small, steepled lantern or bellcote (see Fig. 2). By the early fifteenth century, the close had earned the name of 'Deademannescroft'.[99] This burial ground is known to lie between what is now Great Sutton Street on the north, and Clerkenwell Road on the south (see also Fig. 3 on p. 48).[100]

The principal route out of the city to this new cemetery was through Aldersgate, up past St Bartholomew's priory and along what is now Goswell Road. The dead could also have been taken via Newgate and Smithfield, and thence up St John Street. It is not clear when the cemetery first began to take burials, but an argument can be made that, despite its considerable extent, it was approaching capacity in the early weeks of 1349. The carts removing the dead from the city must have been numerous indeed. As we shall see, a later emergency cemetery of comparable size at East Smithfield was able easily to contain 2,400 burials, a figure which could have been achieved by a rate of some forty burials each day in November and December. Such a rate accords well with the situation described at the beginning of the plague by Robert of Avesbury, who noted that 'on the same day, 20, 40 or 60 bodies, and on many occasions many more, might be committed for burial together in the same pit'.[101] The figure also corresponds with the (later) events described in Tournai when the plague hit that city in 1349. There, 'every day the dead were carried into churches, now five, now ten, now fifteen. And in the church of St Brice, sometimes 20 or 30.'[102] Placing such figures in context,

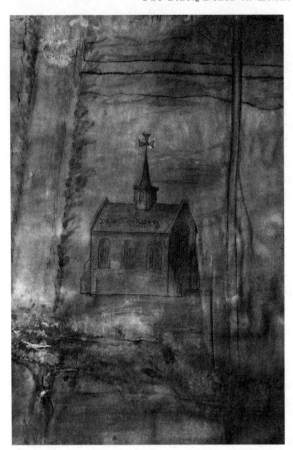

Fig. 2 The Pardon chapel and part of the churchyard established by Bishop Stratford, as drawn in the sixteenth century. The road on the left is St John Street and the linear feature to the right of the chapel is the water supply pipe to the later Charterhouse monastery. (NMRC Neg BB98/12775, Crown Copyright)

if London did have 60,000 souls within its walls, in an untroubled year we might expect six burials or less per day across the entire city.[103] This, however, was just the beginning: things were going to get much, much worse.

The king and his treasurer, Bishop William Edington, both remained in London for much of December. They were in the royal chamber in the Tower of London on 14 December, when the 'infirm and paralysed' John Offord, Archbishop-elect of Canterbury, took the oath of fealty for the temporalities of the Archbishopric,[104] and the king was in Westminster from before 28 December through to January. They were therefore very well placed to witness the unfolding catastrophe. On 1 January 1349 Edward was compelled to write to Edington, cancelling the planned Parliament formally. The letter addressed a 'certain parliament of ours concerning great and weighty matters … and the state of our realm, at Westminster on Monday after St Hilary [19 January]', to which it was intended that the bishop would appear in person with the other prelates and magnates. It explained:

since a sudden and deadly plague has arisen there and round about, and has so grown in strength that men are fearful to go there safely during this time, we have, for these and other obvious reasons, ordered that the said parliament be prorogued [until 27th April 1349], and for this reason, you should not come there on the Monday.

The letter reiterated instruction that when Parliament did reconvene, the prior of Winchester and the archdeacon were to attend in person, the chapter to send one procurator and the diocesan clergy to send two, and that no excuses would be allowed.[105] The king then left for the Augustinian priory of Merton, 8 miles south-west of the city, to celebrate the Epiphany on 6 January for jousting and games, some of which may have involved a funereal aspect.[106]

It may have been at around this time that accusations of poisoning the water supply of the city were made. Fear of well-poisoning by 'foreigners' and Jews had already gripped European cities and contributed to the dreadful massacres of Jews. England, of course, had no permanent Jewish communities at this time, but it seems probable that other scapegoats were targeted. The Conduit, the principal piped water supply situated in Cheapside, was under the administration of two masters, at this time Robert Fundour and William de St Albans. They raised money from the lease of tankards for collecting the water, and from certain local properties whose rent contributed to the upkeep of leaden pipes extending as far as Westminster and to the conduit house itself. Their accounts, covering a two-year period from November 1348, show that at one specific time, the hefty sum of 32s 2d was spent 'examining the Conduit when it was slandered for poison, by command of the Mayor'.[107] Clearly the supply was found to be clean, and in any event, it would soon become abundantly obvious that the water from the west of the city was not carrying this particular scourge.

The Depths of Despair, January 1349

And there was in those days death without sorrow, marriage without affection, self-imposed penance, want without poverty, and flight without escape.[108]

These words were written by John of Reading, the Westminster monk who witnessed the calamity first-hand, and their brevity exposes the helplessness and horror in the face of the catastrophe far better than could any extended description. The sheer scale of the disaster, becoming clear now to king and commoner alike, must truly have felt like the end of the world. The number of Husting wills, both drawn up and enrolled in January and February, leave no doubt on this. Thirty-eight new wills were compiled in January and a further fifty in February, a monthly rate eighteen times greater than that prior to the outbreak; and four more citizens received personal papal permission to choose confessors,[109] as the wealthier now scrambled to secure and safeguard their inheritances, estates and souls.

One striking aspect of these will-makers is their favouring of the church or churchyard of St Giles Cripplegate as a place of burial at this time. St Giles was the single most popular location within the list of Husting wills written between October 1348 and the end of 1350, with no fewer than thirteen wills specifying burial there (four more even than at St Paul's Cathedral, the next most popular place).[110] All were drawn up between the end of November 1348 and the first week of April 1349, eight being written in the days between 8 January and 8 February 1349; and while this reflects to some degree the cluster of will-making in general in the first three months of the year, the concentration remains very significant. This was not a trade gild concentration, and neither were all the testators parishioners – they came from all across the city. St Giles' power as the patron saint of lepers, beggars, cripples, and of those struck by sudden misery, was surely what drew so many frightened citizens to request their final resting places there. The church clearly had a special recognition in the minds of the beseiged citizens.

An illustration of how suddenly this misery could strike may be provided by a few examples from the wills. On 7 January John Palmer, a shipwright living in an area called Petit Wales on the waterfront near the Tower of London, made his will bequeathing his tenements to his wife Amy, and requesting burial in the churchyard of All Hallows Barking. Within twenty-four hours Amy had drawn up her own will, describing her as 'relict' of John and requesting that her tenements received 'of her late husband' be sold to pay her debts and maintain her son Alan:[111] John had evidently made his will and died within the day. Enrolment of his will was delayed until Amy herself had perished, some time before the end of July 1349.

Stephen de Waltham, a girdler, made his will on 2 February, desiring burial in the churchyard of St Lawrence Jewry and leaving his tenement to his wife Margery, with the remainder of his estate bequeathed to his executor, Ralph Abraham. In the event, it was only Ralph who came to court on 9 February for the probate: Margery had succumbed within a week of her husband's death.[112] Johanna Amyel, daughter of a chandler, made her will on 8 February, wishing burial in the churchyard of St Botolph Aldgate and leaving part of her estate to her sister Cristina. By the time Cristina had drawn up her own will on 13 February, Johanna was already dead, and Cristina was to outlast her sister by less than three days; her will was enrolled on 16 February.[113]

The preparations that people made, most likely in the knowledge that they had already contracted the disease and were doomed to die, are also poignantly visible in the records. Johanna Elys, whose husband had already died, set out her will on 5 February, probably even as she suffered the first agonies of the disease. In it, she attempted to secure the financial future of her son and daughter, Richard and Johanna. She set out a share of tenements in St Bride Fleet Street and St Dunstan in the West between them, and made specific bequests of beds, pots and pans that each child was to receive. Finally, given their minority, she placed them under the guardianship of her own mother. Having done her best for her children, she died less than seventy-two hours later.[114]

In total, eighteen wills were enrolled in the Court of Husting between 20 and 26 January: a figure we might expect to represent a year's sum had been reached in a week. By the end of February a further twenty-two wills had been added to the rolls. Among the dead were the Archdeacon of London, Henry Iddesworth; the rectors of St Margaret Friday Street and of St Mary Woolnoth; Thomas Crosse, the recently appointed dean of St Stephen's Westminster; John Kelleseye, whose wife was to distribute the silver to the poor; and many others. Across the Thames, Lambeth lost its rector, John de Colonia, in February or early March.[115]

As with rich, so with poor. The bishop's manorial court at Stepney sat again on 20 January, some seven weeks after the last session. In those weeks, twenty-seven of the bishop's tenants had died, a rate of two deaths every three days from a single manor. The following court, held just three weeks later, confirmed that a further sixty-one tenant deaths had occurred, indicating that the mortality rate had doubled. Once again, families were hit by multiple deaths, such as the Bischops who lost John, the father, and two of his sons, John and Peter, leaving a sole heir, William.[116] It is clear that by the end of January the toll was becoming unmanageable, even with the new Pardon cemetery set aside by Bishop Stratford. Boccaccio's *Decameron* provides us with a vivid picture of the nightmare; Florence might easily be London in this passage:

> the majority of [the poor] were constrained, either by their poverty or the
> hope of survival, to remain in their houses. Being confined to their own parts
> of the city, they fell ill in their thousands, and since they had no one to assist
> them or attend to their needs, they inevitably perished almost without excep-
> tion. Many dropped dead in the open streets, both by day and by night, whilst

a great many others, though dying in their own houses, drew their neighbours' attention to the fact more by the smell of their rotting corpses than by any other means.[117]

London has no such record, but the Register of Charterhouse, an early sixteenth-century document building on fourteenth-century records, describes how the 'violent pestilence killed such a great multitude that the existing cemeteries were insufficient for which reason very many were compelled to bury their dead in places unseemly and not hallowed or blessed; for some, it was said, cast corpses into the river'.[118] There is corroboration for such desperate acts as this: at Avignon early in 1348, so great were the numbers of dead that the Pope blessed the waters of the Rhone so that bodies carried by the river might receive at least a minimal religious ceremony.[119]

Some sort of solution to the problem posed by unburied corpses was urgently required, and it came from one of the king's most valued servants and military men during the French campaigns in the 1340s, Sir Walter de Mauny, who was in the city at this time. As well as conducting the truce on behalf of the king, he had been a prominent knight on the field, an admiral of the king's fleet, and a trusted servant of Edward in many other matters. For his services he had been summoned to Parliament as a baron from 1347. He was, in addition, the marshal of the Marshalsea prison throughout spring and summer 1349.[120]

Whether through piety or through recognition of the peril arising from numerous unburied corpses, de Mauny determined in January to greatly increase the size of Stratford's cemetery to the north of the city. His first action was to obtain some land, undertaken between the foundation of the bishop's cemetery in December 1348 and January 1349. He leased from St Bartholomew's hospital 'an enclosed space for the purpose of a burying ground for those who had died of pestilence, called the Spitell Croft at 12 marks per year', with the understanding that he should be granted full possession when he could provide the hospital with property of equal value in exchange.[121] Later, in de Mauny's own words to the Pope in August 1352, evidence that the cemetery was assigned a specific role comes to light. The knight stated that 'during the epidemic in England, he dedicated a place near London for a cemetery of poor strangers (*peregrinorum*) and others … and built there a chapel with the licence of the ordinary [Bishop Stratford]'.[122] The use of the term *peregrinorum* is significant, since it indicates that the people for which this cemetery was established were not citizens, but were more likely the poor who had flocked to the city out of desperation or false hope, or were traders and visitors caught up in the nightmare.

The Register of Charterhouse describes how Bishop Stratford 'assembled a great multitude and with solemn procession came to the cemetery site, dedicating it in the honour of the Holy and Undivided Trinity and the Annunciation of Our Lady'.[123] The precise date of this consecration is unclear, but the cemetery was already functioning by 26 January 1349, when de Mauny obtained a licence from the king to provide support for its religious oversight. The licence allowed him to pass properties to the value of £100 yearly to a proposed chapel, 'within the place newly dedicated for the burial of the dead by the city of London'.[124] Geoffrey le Baker's chronicle tells us that the name of the cemetery was Newchurchehawe and that the house of religion to be founded there was specifically for the burial of the dead.[125] In Robert of Avesbury's eyes, the cemetery was of considerable importance for the management of the plague victims. He reported that between Candlemas (2 February) and Easter (12 April), 'more than 200 bodies were carried to the cemetery for burial almost every day',[126] perhaps some 14,000 over the seventy-day period described. How such numbers were transported to the cemetery is not specified in any document, but the chronicler William of Dene's graphic account of matters at Rochester no doubt stood for London too. He reported:

> this mortality devoured such a multitude of both sexes that no-one could be found to carry the corpses of the dead to burial but men and women carried the bodies of their own little ones to church on their shoulders and threw them into mass graves from which arose such a stink that it was barely possible for anyone to go past a churchyard.[127]

Aldersgate must have witnessed a grim procession indeed passing beneath its arch, with a new corpse emerging from the stricken city on average every five minutes. The cemetery now lies under Charterhouse Square and the site of Charterhouse (see Fig. 3).[128]

The enormity of the disaster meant that some breakdown in administration was inevitable. On 26 January the King's Bench, the principal court delivering the king's justice and held in Westminster Palace, was suspended. Edward wrote to his justices in no uncertain terms:

> Mindful of the terrible pestilence of vast deadliness, daily increasing in the city of London and neighbouring parts, we do not wish any danger to threaten you, your serjeants, clerks and the other officers of the said bench, nor the people transacting their business there. With the assent of bishops, earls, barons and others of our council staying at Langley, we have given instruction that all

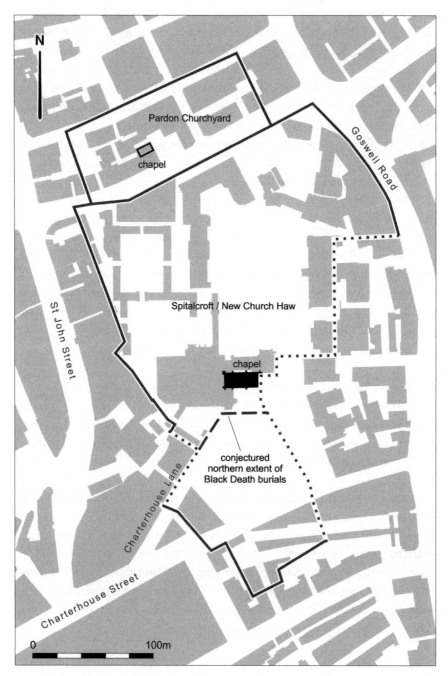

Fig. 3 The disposition of lands set aside for Bishop Stratford's Pardon churchyard, and Walter de Mauny's Newchurchehawe (after Barber and Thomas 2002, fig. 15). The conjectured extent of burials proposed is based on negative evidence from a number of excavations in the cemetery area. (Courtesy of MoLA)

... pleas before you at the bench are to be held over from now until the quin-
dene of [the fortnight following] Easter [27 April] ... We wish you to institute
a procedure regarding these writs to be returned at the bench so that hearings
may take place without discontinuation or delay.[129]

In fact, the King's Bench was not to meet again until Michaelmas 1349.

February 1349

If administration was under pressure, the evidence is very scant for any resultant breakdown of law and order. The only direct example arises from a case
before the court of Possessory Assizes, itself closed after August 1348 until
late 1349. This court, whose purpose was to investigate allegations of unlaw-
ful dispossession of property, heard a case on 7 November 1349 relating to
events in February. One Robert de Walcote claimed that on 23 February five
men had ejected him from his rightful hold of three tenements in the parish
of St Leonard Candlewick Street by force of arms. The case proceeded until
May 1350 when the court found for Robert; the defendants were imprisoned and forced to pay 100s damages. Two further cases of dispossession
during the plague months (on 30 April and 25 May) were also heard, but
these did not involve allegations of violence.[130]

In contrast to this meagre evidence, it is quite clear that attempts were
made to continue the normal business of managing city and realm as far
as was possible. The mayor and city aldermen did continue to meet, to
hear pleas and to enrol charters and wills at Husting (see Chapter 3). On
14 February eight of the elected shearmen brought the ordinances for the
government of their guild before the mayor, though six of those eight were
dead or missing within weeks, as noted on the Letter Book itself.[131] The
infirm Archbishop-elect of Canterbury, John de Offord, had put before the
city new ordinances, dated 13 January, for the future management of the
leper hospital of St Giles to the west of the city.[132] Manorial courts within
the vicinity of London were not abandoned. The court at Stepney met on
10 February and reported a further sixty-one deaths in the three weeks
since 20 January. The manor's estimated toll for the whole of February –
an extraordinary seventy-five deaths – was to be the highest during the
outbreak, the plague peaking in the smaller vills making up the manor as
much as six weeks earlier than in the city itself. Similarly, in the much
smaller manor of Vauxhall, the court recorded eleven deaths between
1 January and 11 February.[133]

Commerce also continued at significant levels; for example, between 28 January and 5 February, the collectors in the Port of London paid, on behalf of the king, a total of £517 7s 9½d for 388 sacks and 1 stone (over 63 tons) of wool shipped from King's Lynn to the city by the men of nine different merchants, several of them London woolmongers.[134] Wine too continued to flow through the city. A curious case illustrates both the trade and the continuing determination to regulate it despite the plague. Guilliottus de Gaignebien and Anthony Macenoie, Basque wine merchants from Placencia, had set out from Lisbon with 261 tuns of wine in late January or early February. While awaiting fair weather in a port in Brittany, their ships had been impounded illegally by Thomas Dagworth, Edward's administrator for that region. Dagworth confiscated the wine and had it shipped to English ports, including London, for sale for his own profit. The outraged merchants appealed to the king, who on 12 February commanded the sheriffs of London to organise a search of all wine cellars and other wine stores in the city to locate any of the missing wine.[135]

The property market remained active, doubtless buoyed up to some degree by the implementation by executors of enrolled wills or the reorganisation of rental arrangements within families. For example, the cartulary of St John Clerkenwell, the Hospitaller priory adjacent to the Pardon cemetery, recorded among land transactions between its tenants an instance of property-swapping between relatives. A charter dated 19 February 1349 records a grant by Peter atte Gate to his relative, Robert atte Gate, of a tenement worth 12d in rental, lying west of St John Street adjacent to the priory, in the parish of St Sepulchre Newgate. Two days later, Robert re-granted to Peter the same tenement, to hold for life, for nominal payment to Robert and his heirs. Should Peter die, the tenement would revert to Robert.[136] Similarly, on 20 July 1349 Thomas de Salisbury and Alice, his wife, granted houses and a quay on the 'Stonewharf' between Bere Lane and Thames Street (near the Custom House) to John Nott, Peter de Gilnefford and Thomas de Bonwode. On 22 July Nott and Bonewode handed the property back.[137] It may have been the death of Gilnefford, who is absent from the re-grant, that triggered this.

March 1349

In March, the rate at which Londoners were preparing wills increased again: no fewer than eighty-nine were drawn up this month, twelve of them on a single day, the 12th. Over one-quarter of this total were dead before the month was out, and a total of sixty-one wills were enrolled at the Husting court's four dated meetings: 2, 9, 16 and 23 March. However, it is clear that the system for enrolling the wills was beginning to show some sign of strain. Two enrolments, those of Roger Carpenter, a pepperer in St Benet Sherehog parish, and Stephen atte Holte, a timber-monger in St Michael Cornhill, show that the dates they were drawn up actually post-dated, by five and one day respectively, the court at which they were enrolled – an obvious impossibility.[138] It is possible that the will scribes got the dates wrong, it is also possible that there was in fact an additional court held on 30 March, but that the separate dates were not formally entered into the roll as such. Perhaps as experienced clerical staff became victims, they were being replaced by those unused to the standard procedure.

Among the poor tenants of Stepney, the court roll for 19 March 1349 indicates that a total of ninety-two further tenants had died since the previous court on 10 February, bringing the total death toll for the manor to 185 since November. The estimated toll for the whole of March was sixty-six deaths, so while the peak in the manor may have been reached by the end of February, the plague was still almost as deadly through to the beginning of spring.

The impact on families is obvious: victims included five of the atte Walle family, four of the Pod family, three members of the Pentecost family, and a further two Pymmes who had all died in the previous seven weeks. Two of the Cobbe family included one Alexander Cobbe, who was probably the same man as had been elected to represent Portsoken ward on the first Common Council of the city in 1347.[139] The date of death of his colleague on the council, farrier Alexander Mareschal, can be narrowed down by a rare crossover between tenancy records from the manor and Husting will enrolments. Mareschal's Stepney holding was put into the hands of the bishop after 19 March, and his will was enrolled on 23 March, so he must have died between the two dates.[140] No relevant Vauxhall court rolls survive.

With such an elevated mortality rate in the city, the deaths of members from more than one generation within individual free families made the arrangements for passing on inheritances complex. Richard de Shordych had drawn up his will on 10 February and was dead by the beginning of March. We do not know what his profession was, but in the will he left a tenement in St Olave Jewry to his son John, and goods and money to Benedict and Margaret, his other children. Richard's wife Margery had died earlier (at an unknown date) and her family had already inherited property from her; son Benedict had received land in the parish of St Stephen Coleman Street. In the grip of plague, Benedict drew up his own will on 6 March 1349, and was himself dead by the 16th. Father and son appear on the Husting roll almost adjacent. Benedict was obviously one of the executors of his father's will, but had no time at all to accomplish the execution; in his own will he is able only to set aside the land his mother left him for a chantry in St Olave, and to request his master, John Lacer, to act in his stead as executor for his father's undischarged will.[141] John Lacer, in his turn, may well be the man of that name whose own will was drawn up in April 1349, and who died by the beginning of May.[142] If so, property was passing within days from father to son to executor to executor's nominee(s); the risks in maintaining a clear trail of ownership are obvious.

The emergency cemeteries founded by Bishop Stratford and Walter de Mauny also feature for the first time in the wills of Londoners in March 1349: they had very rapidly become incorporated into the civic landscape. That of Gerard Larmurer was drawn up on 3 March. He probably lived in the parish of St Bride Fleet Street, and made arrangements to leave his estate to his wife Eustacia, and Ralph and Isabella, his children, with a clause that if no heir was forthcoming from them, he would:

> leave and ordain that the said possession shall descend to the new chapel of the Blessed Virgin Mary outside Aldersgate, to have and to hold in perpetuity, on condition that the … chapel be required … to maintain a priest who shall celebrate mass in perpetuity for the souls of my father and mother, my ancestors and all the faithful departed.[143]

This is the earliest reference to the chapel that Walter de Mauny had set out to build in his extended cemetery for poor strangers, and indicates that, at the least, groundwork or other preparatory activities for the chapel, such as stockpiling building materials, were under way, and that some citizens at least were aware of de Mauny's project. The formal foundation ceremony for the chapel took place some three weeks after this will was made, according to the Charterhouse Register. On the Annunciation of Our Lady (25 March) 1349, the Bishop of London:

> with the Mayor of the City and the sheriffs, as well as the more eminent citizens who are called aldermen, and many others, nearly all barefooted and with a most devout procession, went to the said cemetery, and there the bishop celebrated and preached a solemn sermon to the people … On the same day the Mayor laid the foundation of the chapel.[144]

Such a procession, leading as it would have done from the Guildhall itself, via the cathedral and then out through Aldersgate towards the cemetery, would have been quite an occasion at the height of the crisis, and would certainly have served to give hope to the beleaguered citizens. The chapel survived to become the church of the later Carthusian monastery of Charterhouse and its site was excavated in the early 1950s. It was originally a stone building set out on a rectangular plan of four or possibly five bays, measuring approximately 30m in length by 10m wide. Evidence for a dais was found at its eastern end. The walls were of chalk and ragstone, common building materials at this time.[145]

The West Smithfield cemeteries were evidently still insufficient to cope with the numbers of dead; more space for burial was required and consequently a third cemetery was established, again just beyond the walls, on the eastern side of the city at Tower Hill. The origin of this cemetery is somewhat less clear than that in West Smithfield, but it must have been founded just a little after. The story begins several years prior to the plague's appearance, with the decision of one John Cory to acquire land on Tower Hill. John Cory was a royal servant with particular skills in numbers and accounts. He was collecting debts for the Crown in Exeter in 1341, and became surveyor of weights and measures for Devon, Somerset and Dorset between 1342 and 1344. By May 1346 he was working for the Black Prince in Devon, and in 1349 he was appointed as the prince's Attorney General in Chancery, the Exchequer and before the justices of both Benches. He had a house in the parish of St Michael Queenhithe by 1353.

There may be reason to believe that Cory was acquiring land on Tower Hill on behalf of the king for the foundation of a monastery on the site. The earliest such acquisition was in May 1346, of a brewery owned by Richard le Botoner, a London pepperer.[146] The brewery was situated between the road on Tower Hill on the west and a field called 'Horselegfurlong' on the east. Acquisition of similar tenements and lands on Tower Hill, between Hog Street and East Smithfield, continued throughout 1348. However, in 1349, 'at the urging of substantial men of the City', and with the agreement of Nicholas, prior of Holy Trinity priory, Aldgate, Cory asked Bishop Stratford to consecrate part of his holdings, probably the Horselegfurlong field, as a burial ground.[147] The cartulary of the priory indicates that it is this connection that provided the cemetery with its name: the churchyard of the Holy Trinity.

The scale of the cemetery was not that of de Mauny's (see Fig. 4). It measured initially 147 ells by 93 ells on its longest sides – roughly 170m by 107m or about 4 acres in all – and was walled around with an earthen bank. Exactly when it was consecrated is not stated, but a priory document of the mid-1360s cites the inadequacy of existing space for the burial of victims as the reason,[148] so it was most probably after November 1348, and the best guess is January or February 1349, immediately after Cory obtained the field, and perhaps just a few weeks later than de Mauny's cemetery.

By Easter Sunday, 12 April, a chapel was either planned or being built, since the will of Andrew Cros, a fishmonger, drawn up on that date, specified his wish to 'leave my body to be buried in the cemetery of Holy Trinity next to the Tower of London … [with] 5s for the works of the chapel there [*operi capelle ibidem*]'. Similarly, the will of Johanna, wife of John de Colchester, also a fishmonger, requested her body 'to be buried in the new cemetery of Holy Trinity next to the Tower of London … [leaving] 20s for the works of the chapel of the said cemetery'. This will was made out on 22 April.[149]

The identity of the 'substantial men of the City' who saw the need for additional burial space is something of a mystery. The term does not suggest the mayor and aldermen, who would have been easy to define, but rather a syndicate of influential citizens. One of the parcels of land acquired by Cory came from Thomas de Cotyngham,[150] perhaps the same Thomas Cotyngham who was one of the king's advisers and who would receive the great seal on the order of the king following the death of John de Offord in May 1349. Other prominent Londoners with links to the site include Andrew Cros, who willed burial in the cemetery and whose kinswoman, Helena Cros, was to pass further adjacent lands to Cory in 1350[151] suggesting family connections; Johanna de Colcestre, among the earliest recorded to have willed burial in April; and finally, William de Shordych, a goldsmith, whose will, made in May 1349, named Prior Nicholas as the guardian of his son.[152] In any event, the first three months of the year thus saw two new churches rising to serve the city over the coming months, specifically dedicated to the salvation of the souls of plague victims through the intercession on the one hand of the Virgin Mary, with her particular power to avert the wrath of God, and on the other the Holy Trinity.

The scale of the pestilence continued to interfere with the business of running the kingdom and the city. On 10 March the king accepted the fact that his postponement of the January Parliament would effectively have to be indefinite. He wrote:

> Whereas lately, by reason of the deadly pestilence then prevailing, we caused the Parliament that was summoned to meet at Westminster on the Monday after the Feast of St Hilary to be prorogued until the quinzaine of Easter next – and because the aforesaid pestilence is increasing with more than its usual severity, in Westminster and in the City of London and the surrounding districts, whereby the coming of the magnates and other of our faithful lieges to that place at this time would probably be too dangerous – for this, and for

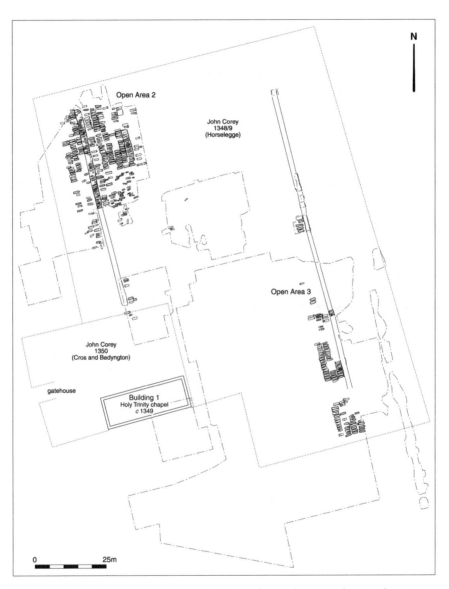

Fig. 4 The layout of the East Smithfield churchyard of the Holy Trinity, showing the west and east burial zones and the probable location of the chapel and later gatehouse. (Courtesy of MoLA)

certain other obvious reasons we have thought fit to postpone the said Parliament until we shall issue further summons.[153]

What the king meant by 'usual severity' is unclear. It may indicate the frequency with which late winter or spring pestilences occurred in London, or it may indicate that London was considered to be especially hard hit in the current outbreak. Royal business that did carry on in London at this time included the undertaking of Inquisitions Post Mortem, surveys undertaken after the death of a tenant in chief to establish the estates held and the rightful successor(s). The pestilence dramatically increased this workload nationally, and at least one survey, of the Middlesex lands of one Roger Bedyngfield, was held at West Smithfield on 11 March. Later examples included that of Hugh le Despenser on 22 April 1349, conducted by John Lovekyn as mayor and escheator for the city.[154]

Evidence of the need to replace royal officials (though not categorically due to plague losses) can be seen in the king's grant for life to Richard de Hame of the position of surveyor of the Thames between the city and Staines,[155] and the appointment of a new clerk of works and a new controller of works at Westminster and the Tower.[156] The work of the mint did not cease during the crisis; indeed work on Edward's new coin types remained an important priority. On 24 March, the day before the commonalty of London were to go barefoot to de Mauny's new chapel site, Edward issued an indenture to three Italians – John Donati, Philip John de Neir of Florence and Benedict Isbare of Lucca – to make three types of gold coin in the Tower of London. The largest was the gold noble, then worth 6s 8d and calculated at 42 pieces to each pound weight of gold; there was also a half and a quarter gold piece, and a range of silver coins.[157] The indenture agreement was witnessed by several London merchants, who clearly had a direct interest in the issue of this new coin, including John de Colewell, a wealthy mercer, and Robert de Shordich, a goldsmith.

The mayor and sheriffs, who had not met to consider pleas since September 1348, met once in March, showing that the business of justice continued at least in some form in the city despite the severity of the crisis. One John Shonke of Lesnes in Kent had been confined in Newgate prison in connection with an unpaid debt to Robert Cros, a fishmonger's son (and presumably a relative of the Cros family involved in the land transfers for the East Smithfield cemetery). Claiming that he had already paid off the debt, Shonke sought justice in the court. Cros denied that payment had been made but a jury found for the plaintiff, who received 100s damages, while his creditor replaced him in gaol.[158] The civic authorities, like the king, found need

to replace lost officers, and on 20 March Thomas de Neuport was admitted serjeant of the chamber of the Guildhall by the mayor, aldermen and
commonalty. He was dead within a month.[159] The trade guilds, too, must
have been very badly hit; certainly of three bailiffs of the Weavers' Company
elected in November 1348, Richard Horewode was dead by 4 March, and
John de Whitefeld's will, dated 19 March, was proved just a few weeks later.[160]

April 1349

In the city, the plague undoubtedly reached its height in April, some
six weeks after it peaked in the nearby manor of Stepney. No fewer than
104 wills were drawn up during this one month, seven on Easter Sunday
alone (12 April), suggesting that many, if not most, wealthy Londoners were
now convinced that they could no longer expect to survive and thus had to
make preparations for their death; it also implies that perhaps spoken (or nuncupative) wills were now considered of little use since those to whom they
were addressed had just as much chance of perishing. Insights into the development of contingency tactics can be gained from these wills. Many citizens
were now not only worried about their own survival, but also that of those
who they may appoint to look after their offspring should the worst happen.

David de Kyngestone, in his will of 3 April, bequeathed his properties in
the parish of St Margaret Lothbury to his children, Simon and Johanna. He
appointed as guardians two men, John Lucas for his son and John de Herlawe
for his daughter. Colewell (also known as Coterel), the mercer who witnessed the indenture of the Italian coiners, made his will on the same date,
and in it appointed two other mercers as guardians of his children, Adam
Fraunceys to Thomas and Hugh de Wychyngham for his daughter Johanna,
leaving his wife as guardian of his second son John. Isabella Godchep, in
her will drawn up on Easter Sunday, appointed multiple guardians for her
grandson.[161] By such tactics, the chances of at least one child retaining an
adult carer of the parents' choice must have been greatly enhanced.

Such care was not necessarily confined to immediate family. John de
Mymmes, an image-maker (*ymaginour*), in his will on 19 March 1349, left
properties in St Mildred Poultry to his wife Matilda and two daughters,
Alice and Isabella, and appointed Roger Osekyn, a pepperer of Bread Street,
to guard Isabella (presumably the younger of the two) should his wife die
before the girl reached maturity. John was dead by 10 April, when Matilda
drew up her own will, but neither Matilda's will nor that of Osekyn (dated
13 April) makes any mention of the daughters. Isabella certainly was alive

(and survived to full age[162]), but Matilda chose instead to leave a bequest to one William, her apprentice image-maker. He was to receive the best third of the tools and copies for picture-making, and was to be sent to work under Brother Thomas de Alsham at Bermondsey Abbey near Southwark for three years,[163] presumably to further his skills. We do not know how William fared, although it would be satisfying to discover that the convent at Bermondsey had delighted in some of his images; Matilda herself followed her husband, probably one daughter and Osekyn to the grave in May.

Forced to take account of an extraordinary, rapidly evolving situation, some of these wealthier families looked to a central system of security to act as a safety net should their best-laid plans falter. Adam Aspal was a wealthy skinner with properties in Bread Street, Cornhill and Billingsgate. He left these to his wife Auncillia in his will dated 15 April, with some additional estate to his sons John and Richard and his daughter Juliana, probably knowing he was dying. The will contained the prescient clause that Auncillia's property should be sold after her death to pay Adam's debts: Auncillia wrote her own will just six days later, and she too was dead days after making it. The key fact in her will is that she had previously agreed to act as guardian for the children of a fishmonger, John de Neuport, but wished now to pass money received for this purpose (presumably from Neuport) into the care of the Chamberlain of the Guildhall, at this time one Thomas de Maryns, until the children came of age.[164] Such wards of the city could then be passed on to suitable guardians chosen by the mayor and aldermen, and an example of this is to be found in the City Letter Books. On 22 April the mayor and aldermen committed to one William Oyldebeof of Colmworth, Bedfordshire, the guardianship of three sons of Londoner Hugh le Plasterer. Possibly this meant that the young boys, Robert aged 12, John aged 9 and Thomas aged 6, started a new life away from the city.[165]

Some who had appointed guardians returned to wills drawn up earlier to make amendments in the light of the disaster, and one in particular provides a sense of pessimism about the likely outcome. William Hanhampsted, a pepperer in the parish of St Antonin, had drawn up his will in January 1349, appointing his wife and eldest son as guardians over the other five children. On 28 April, however, he added a codicil to the will stating that should his wife and children all die within one year of his own death, the Church was to inherit his entire estate for pious uses.[166]

His pessimism was only partly realised: we learn from the City Letter Books that the plague claimed him, his wife and one daughter, but all three sons and two other daughters survived at least as far as 1353. His wife, Agnes, provides evidence of wills made and proved before an ecclesiastical court, but not subsequently enrolled in Husting. Her will was dated 29 May (by which time William was already dead) and endorsed before Roger de Kempele, commissary-general of Ralph, Bishop of London. Her pessimism is also apparent, as she bequeaths a sum to Alice, her servant, 'or whoever else shall nurse her son John until he is weaned'.[167]

Even unborn children were remembered within bequests, such as that of Thomas atte Vyne, who left 'to John, Thomas, Geoffrey, and Andrew his sons, and to his child *en ventre sa mere,* bequests of money, silver cups and brass pots … [and] … the reversion of all rents within and without the gate where his aforementioned mother resides'.[168] This was not an exclusive feature of the pestilence, but of a total of fifty-five examples from all Husting wills between 1259 and 1688, five fell within the months of November 1348 through to April 1349 (see Fig. 15 on p. 163).

Guardians might be used to attempt to safeguard establishments as well as people. In 1329 the very wealthy mercer William of Elsing had founded near Cripplegate a new hospital of St Mary for 100 blind men, and the project was still in development when the plague struck, since Augustinian canons had yet to be installed to run it. Elsing made his will on 23 March 1349 and in it extended the remit to include the 'poor, blind and indigent of both sexes', quite probably recognising a de facto change to the intended foundation situation. For their support he left to the hospital considerable properties in at least eight parishes. Both the hospital and these properties were placed under the guardianship of Elsing's executors until such time as a prior and canons could be elected to take charge.[169]

An increasingly popular form of defence against the effects of plague that comes to light in the wills drawn up in April was that of membership of a religious fraternity. Fraternities were essentially religious societies, more often than not associated with a single trade or craft, and usually focused on a specific church. Their members were drawn from the same middle and upper strata of the city as the Husting will-makers. Membership ensured, among other things, that upon death the affairs of the deceased would be discharged and a suitable funeral would be held with mourners drawn from the fraternity itself. Although a small number existed before 1348, the attractiveness of membership of such bodies at this time of crisis was clear.[170] Thus John de Shenefeld, a tanner, left in his will of 1 April a tenement to the fraternity of the Light of St Mary in the church of St Sepulchre Newgate; William de Flete, a mercer, on 5 April, and Nicholas de Rothe, a salter, on 12 April, left property to the fraternity of Corpus Christi in All Hallows Bread Street. Also on 12 April, Andrew Cros, the fishmonger who willed burial in the new plague cemetery on Tower Hill, left money to the fraternity of St Magnus on Bridge Street. Some bequests were more specific in their aims to support the fraternity's activities. The wealthy goldsmith Simon de Berkyng made his will in January 1349, leaving a mansion to help provide income for the almonry of the fraternity of St Dunstan in the Goldsmithery, presumably a safety net for the fraternity members and their families.[171]

Other notable wills drawn up in April include that of Matilda atte Vigne (dated the 22nd), the widow who had blocked out the light of the queen's tailor the previous September. Matilda had separately applied for papal permission to choose her own confessor in April, or perhaps a little earlier, possibly with her eye on Sir Thomas, chaplain of her own chantry chapel in St Edmund Lombard Street which she had founded over twenty years earlier,[172] to whom she bequeathed 100s and a substantial £20 for him to purchase a 'convenient house'. The remainder of her estate was to go to kinsmen and friends, and especially to her executors Matilda Ram, her niece, and John Charteney. Her plans for departing this life appear to have been compromised by the plague in both the short and the longer term. She was dead by 4 May (when the will was proved), just days before papal permission for a confessor arrived on the 7th.[173] Her will remained unexecuted for at least three years, since Charteney was, in his own will of August 1352, forced to admit that he had not discharged his duty as executor, passing the entire burden of administration over to Matilda Ram.[174]

Geoffrey Chaucer's family, living in a tenement in Thames Street, was also caught up in the plague in April. Chaucer himself would have been about 9 when the plague struck and, while he survived, Thomas Hayron, half-brother to Geoffrey's father John, made his will on 7 April and was dead before 4 May. John was Hayron's executor, so the two must have been close. Richard Chaucer, his step-grandfather, wrote his will on 12 April, and died in July 1349.[175] Finally, William de Thorneye, John Chaucer's other half-brother, was also dead before the end of July 1349 (see below). It is therefore unsurprising that the plague had a significant impact on the youngster and would resurface in his writing: it is in *The Pardoner's Tale* that Death is characterised as a 'secretive thief, a pestilence who hath a thousand slayn'.

In a rare exception to the norm, one set of wills indicates where a victim died. John Dallyngge was a mercer living in the parish of St Michael Bassishawe. He made his will on 6 April, leaving his tenement to his son, also called John. The father died before 20 May, the date that the son made his own will. In the latter, John requested that the tenement 'in which his father died' be sold to pay his debts and for pious purposes. Neither will was proved in Husting until November, again illustrating the lag between death and enrolment.[176]

Though no will survives, we know that the prior of Westminster Abbey, one Simon de Harmondesham, also perished at the beginning of April. A hitherto-unknown monk called Simon de Langham was swiftly elected in his place, but was to spend less than seven weeks in office before being elevated to the position of abbot – such were the opportunities that accompanied this extraordinary death rate.[177] Similar events were occurring in St Paul's Cathedral as canons succumbed and were replaced. On 7 May John Cok was granted the prebendary of Finsbury on account of the death of Thomas de Asteley, notwithstanding Cok's existing position of treasurer of the cathedral.[178]

While so many wills were being drawn up in April, none were enrolled in the Husting as the court did not sit in this month. Ecclesiastical probates were being heard, however. John de Warefeld, a corn-dealer, made his will on 13 March. On it appears a memorandum showing that it was proved on 17 April before the Archdeacon of London.[179] Similarly, the will of William of Elsing, the hospital founder already mentioned (mislabelled Thomas[180]), has a note indicating probate by William Bordesleye, the Bishop of London's commissary-general, on 3 April 1349; both enrolments had also to wait until 4 May for enrolment in Husting.

Many wills made during the plague were, of course, not presented to the court of Husting. Only a few of these survive, such as that of Walter Cobbe, a citizen and butcher, dated probably 5 December 1348 and proved at the Commissary Court on 6 April 1349, requesting burial in the churchyard of St Botolph Aldgate.[181] Incidental references confirm the former existence of others. On 24 August 1350, during a guardianship hearing for William, son of William Bendebowe, an extract was presented of the father's will dated 21 April 1349 and proved in the court of the Archdeacon of London on 18 May.[182]

To gauge how many people were dying at this appalling height of the disaster, we must look forward to those wills that were enrolled in May, once this backlog had been cleared. The total, 121, was the highest at any time during the 1349 plague. Examining the distribution curve of enrolments through the duration of the plague, we may reasonably presume that a majority of those wills, perhaps seventy, were of April's victims alone. This figure represented over forty times the average monthly death rate recorded by enrolments across the decade before 1348. If extended to all inhabitants of a city of 60,000 souls, this would produce a mortality rate very much in line with the claims made by Robert of Avesbury of over 200 burials daily between February and April in the West Smithfield cemetery alone.

Outside the city walls, in the manor of Stepney, the number of deaths was now diminishing, albeit slowly. On 22 April deaths recorded in the court rolls numbered sixty since 19 March,[183] with a resulting estimated toll of forty-five for the whole of April, among whom were four members of the Hemmyngs family.

The dead and their resting places had already achieved prominence in the minds of the living, references to the new cemeteries near Aldersgate and on Tower Hill appearing in wills as often as most parish churches. However, the scale of the mortality continued to impact on Londoners, and a new name was coined for part of the cemetery at St Paul's Cathedral. William de Blithe, a saddler, willed on 16 April to be buried in the 'Pardonchurchehawe' (or Pardon churchyard) above the 'tumulus' of Ralph, his father.[184] Later wills stipulating the same graveyard make it entirely clear that this was directly north of the cathedral church and not a confusion with the new Pardon churchyard in Clerkenwell. The great cathedral cemetery had been used for the burial of Londoners for centuries, but had never before been so referred, and so a link to the pestilence seems certain. How it had gained this new name is not clear, but it may be that the pardons offered to citizens as reward for their involvement in the weekly processions instigated at the start of the plague provided the basis for it. Elsewhere in villages near to London, some parish cemeteries were enlarged, no doubt to accommodate the dead of these rural hinterland settlements; one of these was Chiswick (about 9 miles to the west of the city), where on 22 April the king licensed John de Bray, a Chiswick resident, to provide half an acre of land to the dean and chapter of St Paul's in their capacity as parsons.[185]

Such a death rate cannot but have impacted on daily life in the city. It comes as little surprise, therefore, that on 8 April the king wrote to John Lovekyn, Mayor of London, about the state of the streets, in unequivocal language. He ordered that 'human faeces and other filth lying in the streets and lanes of that city and its suburbs should be removed with all speed to places far distant', and that the mayor should 'cause the city and suburbs to be cleaned from all odour and to be kept clean as it used to be in the time of preceding mayors, so that no greater cause of mortality may arise from such smells'. The city and suburbs, 'under the mayor's care and rule, are so foul by the filth thrown out of the houses by day and night into the streets and lanes … that the air is infected, and the city is poisoned' – a situation which in the king's eyes clearly aggravated the 'mortality by the contagious sickness which increases daily'.[186] Carters and rakers, those whose job it was to clean rubbish and ordure off the streets, did not make enough money to claim an enrolment of their wills in the Husting; there is therefore no indication of the numbers killed off by the plague. But it is clear from the complaint that the service they provided was one which plague had swept aside.

Sanitation remained important to the citizens themselves, even at this dire time. The will of goldsmith John de Walpol, drawn up just a few days before the king's commandment, left his daughter Margery a fine house in the parish of All Hallows Bread Street, but specified that when the latrine situated between the house and a neighbour's dwelling became full, the soil should be carried to the Thames for disposal.[187]

Not only were the carters decimated, but the court roll from Stepney manor indicates that by Easter 1349, the ale-tasters (effectively responsible for the quality control of ale sold in the city) in Stratford, Aldgate Street and Holywell Street were reported to be dead,[188] and we can readily imagine the impact on other trades, crafts and services vital to the basic functioning of the city. April was to prove difficult for city administration in other ways, too. Thomas Maryns, the long-serving chamberlain of London, became a victim of the plague. He made his will on 22 April, then on the 23rd, and with the assent of the mayor and city recorder, took care of outstanding business while he still could; certainly farming out the office of bailiff of Southwark to Harlewyn de Honyngtone for a term of two years at an annual payment to the city of £10 10s. His death was recorded two days later.[189] A new serjeant of the chamber at the Guildhall, Antony de Grenewych, was admitted on 20 April, indicating that the previous incumbent had lasted less than a month.[190] The royal infrastructure sustained losses, too: Thomas de Clopton, keeper of the Great Wardrobe, was certainly alive in March 1349, and equally certainly dead by June.[191] He was an elderly man, but plague was the probable cause.

The Onslaught Weakens, May 1349

During May there were a number of indications that the potency of the plague had begun to diminish. Firstly, the number of wills being drawn up dropped considerably to fifty-six, still a very high rate but just over half the previous month's tally and the beginning of a downward trend which was to continue through into the following year. Secondly, it seems that the number of enrolments was also dropping. While May actually saw the great-est number of enrolments (121), this, as has been stated, covered both April and May deaths: the actual figure for May itself was probably in the region of fifty. This diminution of the plague's effects may have been apparent to eye-witnesses and chroniclers of the time. Certainly Robert of Avesbury con-sidered that the 'plague ceased in London with the coming of the grace of the Holy Spirit [31 May]',[192] and while a complete cessation cannot be substantiated through analysis of the evidence from wills for subsequent months, a clear change in language in reference to the plague can be detected from mid-June onwards.

The plague's impact on the churches and religious houses of London was becoming quite clear by this time, both through records of the houses themselves and through the numerous presentations made to churches to fill vacancies left by deaths. Of the monasteries in the London region, Westminster Abbey was particularly sorely affected. Between March and May 1349, Abbot Simon Bircheston, probably the infirmarer John de Ryngestede, and as many as twenty-six other monks were killed. Bircheston, who died in the abbey's manor house at Hampstead on 15 May, was buried in the cloister near the chapter house door with the epitaph:

Simon of Bercheston, venerable abbot,
His merits forever proclaiming his name:
Now supported by the prayers of his brethren,
May this blessed father now flourish with the kind Fathers
    in the presence of God.[193]

A large black slab in the cloister walk is reputed to cover the remains of the other plague victims, though neither memorial can now be identified on the ground. The religious were, of course, not the only victims. William Isyldon made his will on 24 April in his 'hostel within the close of St Bartholomew the Great', so presumably he was a corrodian or guest; he perished by the beginning of June.[194]

The secular clergy were perhaps even more at risk. Westminster Abbey (along with other religious houses) had a right to present rectors and vicars to a number of churches in the city and surrounding area, but since Abbot Langham's election was not to be confirmed by the Pope until July, this responsibility fell instead to the king. Thus, at St James Garlickhythe, Rector John de Carshalton's will was enrolled on 4 May, and a week later the king presented William de Appleton to the church as his replacement. He further presented John de Methelwold at St Clement Eastcheap on 8 May, and Peter Grevet at St Bride Fleet Street a day later.[195]

Another great Benedictine house which had rights of presentation to London churches, St Albans, had suffered losses on a similar scale to those of Westminster, its abbot having died on 12 April. The king was obliged to present on the abbey's behalf John de Colston to the city church of St Michael Wood Street on 11 May, and William de Kelm to St Peter Westcheap on 1 June.[196] Other parish losses are indicated by the king's presentation on

13 May of John Jevcok to the vicarage of St Alphege, Greenwich, just down the Thames, and the will of John Sonday, rector of St Mary Woolchurch, enrolled on 4 May.[197] St Paul's Cathedral was also hit, as shown by the Pope's appointment of at least two replacement canons: on 13 April Roger Holm replaced Henry Iddesworth as a prebendary (though of which prebend is not clear); and on 7 May, at Edward's request, John Cok, the treasurer of London, replaced Thomas de Astelle.[198] Andrew de Offord was also granted papal confirmation of his role as the new Archdeacon of Middlesex replacing Iddesworth.[199]

All of London's hospitals are likely to have been badly affected by the plague, given their particular responsibilities towards the poor and the sick of the city. Certainly at St Thomas, Southwark, so many brethren had been killed by the end of May that William Edington, Bishop of Winchester, appealed to the Pope for his permit for the house to elect Walter de Marlow as prior, despite the fact that the latter was illegitimate. The permission was granted on 14 June.[200] At the leper house of St James Westminster, the warden and all the brothers and sisters were killed except for William de Weston, who was made master in May and his position ratified by the king in July.[201]

Bequests in wills to hospitals, though common prior to the arrival of the pestilence, must have taken on an increased importance during its visitation, as a result of the combination of high mortality among the staff and hugely increased loading of the destitute, displaced and sick, and are numerous in the Husting will rolls for the months of the crisis. Examples include William de Rothyng (will dated 1 May), who left money for keeping lamps burning before the sick at St Thomas, Southwark; a substantial tenement in the parish of St Martin Vintry, left by John Foxton (will of 8 May), to provide support for the weak and infirm lying in St Mary Spital; and intriguingly, the will of Joanna Youn (dated 11 May), leaving property in the parish of St Botolph Billingsgate to the priory of Holy Trinity Aldgate specifically for medicines.[202] This is the only specific reference to medicinal care during the plague so far located, underscoring the reliance on spiritual protection that prevailed at the time.

That medicines continued to be used within the infirmary at Westminster Abbey seems certain. Thomas de Walden, a city apothecary and sometime Chamberlain of the Guildhall, was successful in chasing debts incurred by the abbey infirmarer for prescription before September 1349 and again in 1350. Indeed, the infirmarer who received these payments was none other than John of Reading, the chronicler of the plague itself. The infirmarers' accounts for the years 1348–50 sadly do not survive, so we do not know what kinds of medicines were brought to bear on the plague.[203] London citizens did not, however, found any hospices or hospitals specifically to cater for the plague victims, as did some in European cities. For example, in June 1348, when the plague entered Sansepolcro, in Tuscany, Italy, the lay fraternity of Santa Maria della Misericordia founded a hospital for the victims just beyond the city walls.[204]

Other notable wills made at this time included that of Geoffrey Wychingham, a former mayor of the city and current alderman of the Aldersgate ward. He made his will on 30 April and was dead before 8 June; the register of the Franciscan friary records that his wife's tomb lay in the friary church, but not where he was himself buried.[205] Thomas de Herlawe, an armourer, made his will on 19 May specifying his 'body to be buried in the new burial ground outside Aldersgate in London', and leaving 40*d* to prepare his burial, along with 13*s* 4*d* to the fraternity of the chapel of the church there. He was dead within six days.[206] The will confirms that de Mauny's original aim to establish a college of chaplains within a church in the burial ground had come to fruition, and in a quite extraordinarily short period of four months.

In Stepney, no courts met between 22 April and 6 July, so the measure of mortality can only be inferred from the number of new deaths reported at the latter date. From this, the monthly toll was probably in the region of nineteen deaths, less than half what it had been the previous month, although still significantly high.[207]

It was not just the diminishing rate of both will-making and will enrolment that gave the city a sense that perhaps the worst had passed; a small number of documents refer again to construction work. Following a formal inquisition by John Lovekyn, Mayor of London, and the required payment of 10*s*, the king on 6 May licensed John de Hurleye, Walter de Tyffeld and Matthew le Barbour to assign to Nicholas de Rothewell, parson of All Hallows Bread Street, a plot of land 12ft by 27ft valued at £40 yearly, for the enlargement of the church chancel. Similarly, but on a grander scale, the Carmelite friars of London were licensed to enclose Croker's Lane, running down the entire western side of the friary, from Fleet Street to the river. The plot, measuring 660ft by 12ft, and described as 'of no value', was for the enlargement of their precinct. The licence included permission to sink a well for those living on the lane.[208]

Construction of new houses possibly during, but probably immediately following, the plague is also exemplified by the vivid case brought to court by a tenant of one such house which backed onto a forge and metalworker's workshop. In answer to the tenant's complaints over the height of the forge chimney (12ft lower than customary), the blows of the great hammer (which threatened to shake party walls and buildings down), and the stench of the smoke from seacoal used to fire the furnaces (which penetrated halls and chambers alike), the forge owners sought to dismiss the action, 'because their messuage was built as recently as 1349 [thus later than the original work-shop], is much higher than the house it replaced, and has windows facing the forge, which its predecessors had not'.[209]

Another indicator in support of a gradual amelioration of the crisis may be the evidence of those coming forward to reclaim debts. On 5 May the king's steward, Philip de Weston, ordered the sheriffs of London to seize the assets of the late Henry Wymond, a plague victim, who was in debt to the Crown. The unfortunate Wymond, a woolmonger, had made his will just a week earlier, on 28 April, and had died on the same day as the steward's notice. While he was beyond worry, the mayor and commons of London were perhaps not; by this order, they were cheated of Wymond's bequest to them of a new house in Tower Street, not yet fully completed, near the mansion of Sir John de Cobham.[210] They were, however, also chasing debts themselves, and on 22 May they issued their own order to their serjeant, William de Greyngham, to summon John Anketel, woolman, over a debt of 100 marks due to John Oweyn. Oweyn had died in the plague, but his executors were now wishing to settle matters.

John Anketel could not reply to the summons, having also perished, so his heirs and tenants were called upon to assist in the case. They, in their turn, failed to appear (perhaps as a result of their deaths too), so the court granted execution of the debt and an inquisition was made of the Anketel property. The jurors found that he possessed houses, a brewhouse and shops in the parish of St Mildred Poultry, as well as shops, a brewhouse, solars and ware-houses in the parishes of All Hallows Bread Street and St Mary Magdalene Milk Street, the latter occupied by his widow Agnes.[211] Both cases indicate the level of administrative confusion that must have mired most, if not all, claims for justice and rulings over property ownership and debts during, and immediately following, the plague.

Perhaps more significantly, the Assize of Nuisance, suspended since September 1348, was revived on 28 May and the first case heard is reassur-ingly domestic in nature. One John de Hardyngham, resident of the parish of St Mary Axe, complained that a couple, Henry and Joan atte Wode, and Alice Powel, the widow of a bell-founder, were refusing to rebuild a ruin-ous earthen wall, 80ft long and running along their garden northward to Hardyngham's. Summonsed by the court, Henry and Joan did not appear, but Alice explained that the late Ralph de Blithe, the previous owner of the tenement on which the wall stood (and former husband of Joan atte Wood), leased it in 1332 for twenty years to Alice Powel and her bell-founder husband, John. The condition was that the lessor should repair the wall when necessary, or, if he failed to do so, should deduct from the Powels' rent their reasonable expenses to sort the repairs. The court agreed that this was appropriate, and gave Alice forty days to repair the wall, recovering the costs from her rent to Henry and Joan.[212]

Both the fact that the court met at all and the nature of the dispute would seem to suggest that people now believed that the world might indeed go on. Meetings of some of the London guilds were also resumed at this time. The mercers' guild certainly met in June and July, perhaps for the first time that year.[213] The resumption of more normal business can be detected in evidence from early June of the rearrangement of matters of private debt. One example was that of Simon Rote, a London skinner, who had in 1348 borrowed £200 from the wealthy money-lender David Wollore (Wooller), adding to a prior debt of £100. Rote died at some point in 1349, probably of the plague, but between 10 and 16 June 1349 his widow Isabel, and son Arnold (with his wife), bound themselves for this debt, thus taking on the dead man's obligations.[214]

A final piece of evidence that matters were improving can be seen in the accounts of payments for construction work at the Tower of London and Westminster Palace in the year between September 1348 and 1349.[215] The Cradle Tower foundation stones were delivered on 8 September 1348, so the period covers a specific new building (see Fig. 5). Construction wages were sustained at an average level of £17 per month until late November, when the figure dips sharply during the height of the plague to around £1 12s per month across March, April and May 1349. It rises again in June and July to an average of £15 until December of that year. While this could represent simple variations in the work level required, the timing looks very significant.

If all this evidence points to a lessening of the plague, it was not a cessation, and dark days were set to continue for some time yet. The king's own surgeon, Roger de Heyton, perished on 13 May, a date preserved as a result of an inquisition following dispute over ownership of his house by the gate of the Palace of Westminster.[216] By 18 May, Thomas le Boter, surveyor of the king's works at Windsor and the royal palace at Kennington (near Lambeth), had died, being replaced by John le Peyntour, and by 20 May, John de Sancto Albano, the king's falconer, had also died and been replaced.[217] Late in May, John de Offord, Chancellor of England and Archbishop-elect of Canterbury, was stricken by plague at Tottenham Court. He had been confirmed as archbishop by the Pope, had taken the oaths necessary to serve his king, and was

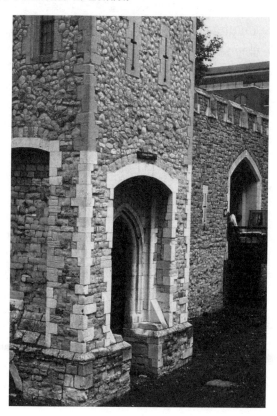

Fig. 5 The Cradle Tower, Tower of London, built during the months of the first outbreak of the Black Death in 1349. (Photograph courtesy of Dr J. Ashbee)

on the cusp of obtaining the additional extensive power and wealth that would flow following his official consecration, despite his age and infirmity. A memorandum to the king recorded his death: 'Be it recorded that Master John de Offord, elect and confirmed to the see of Canterbury, king's chancellor, on 20th May, namely the vigil of the Ascension in this present year, after sunset, departed this life at Totenhall next to London.'[218]

While the Assize of Nuisance had resumed, hearings of Possessory Assizes by the Husting court did not, and would have to wait until 7 November. One of the very first cases to be dealt with referred to events during this period of the plague. One Philip de Herlawe complained that on 25 May four men (Robert de Hatfeld, burreler; Nicholas Hotot, woolman; Roger Hotot and Solomon Faunt) dispossessed him of two messuages in St Mary Woolnoth and St Swithin London Stone. The men denied the charge, Roger and Solomon being represented by an appellant, Alan de Horwode.[219] The date of this is significant, since Philip may well be the son and beneficiary of Thomas de Herlawe, the armourer buried in de Mauny's cemetery in West Smithfield, whose will was proved on the same day as the alleged dispossession.

Of those accused, we do know that Robert de Hatfeld left in his own will in October 1356 a messuage in St Swithin, and that a Nicholas Hotot, woolman, willed to be buried in the church of St Swithin in 1361 during the second pestilence.[220] When the case came to court, it is clear that the confusion lay in the fact that intermediary heirs had also died, and that subsequent holders had potentially disposed of the properties illegally.

June 1349

So began the summer. Will-making in June dropped to levels not seen since the very beginning of the plague: just nine people drew up wills for enrolment in Husting. A dip is also evident in the number enrolled, thirty-one, in the Husting court, but this is due simply to the fact that for one month, from 17 June to 17 July, the court was suspended to permit citizens to attend the Boston fair[221] and, as will be seen, the July figures reflect this.

Of the nine drawn up, the most interesting is that of William de Thorneye. He was a very wealthy pepperer who had held the position of sheriff of London in 1339 and was an alderman in 1342; he was also a half-brother to Geoffrey Chaucer's father, John. He wrote a will and testament, both on 20 June.[222] The will established the disposal of his lands and properties, leaving his young son, John, a shop and tenements in St Mary Aldermary parish, with the remainder going to the nunnery of St Helen's Bishopsgate. The nuns he bound with a complex agreement to establish a chantry for the souls of himself, his family and his kith and kin, requiring them to give security that his bequest would not be used for anything else before both the mayor and aldermen of London, and the justiciar of the King's Bench, Common Pleas or similar. This will was enrolled on 27 July.

The testament set out his wish to be buried in the nunnery church of St Helen's Bishopsgate, near to the tomb of his wife Joanna, and then established the distribution of his moveable goods. He left further money to support perpetual chantries in his parish church, and for a remarkable 10,000 masses to be sung for his soul in various religious houses across the city. Money was also set aside to support the chantries of family and friends in the nunnery church, and to go to numerous religious houses. Among those mentioned in London were: St Helen's Bishopsgate, whose church, dormitory, cloister and other buildings were evidently in need of repair; St Paul's Cathedral; Holy Trinity priory, Aldgate; St Bartholomew Smithfield; St Mary Clerkenwell; and the various hospitals and leper houses around the city.

The will also clearly indicates the level of wealth William was disbursing. No less than £400 in land and tenements was set aside to maintain the chantries, a very considerable sum at the time. Away from London, he left money to the Augustinian houses of Tanridge and Newark in Surrey, and to Thorney Abbey, near his family home in Lincolnshire. At Thorney Abbey he left money to the paupers called 'bedesmen', who dwelled within the monastery, and also to the poor and maim living on the waste ground around its walls. This latter is suggestive of the situation many rural monasteries may have found themselves in as peasants deserted their plague-ridden villages.

Visitors and refugees to London were just as much at risk as the residents. In April 1350 one William de Swynford, accused of 'felonies and trespasses' in Lincoln, was summonsed by the sheriff to give account. On his failure to show, he was threatened with outlawry, but his wife Eleanor pleaded the case, stating that William had died in mid-summer 1349 while visiting William del Chastel in a house in West Smithfield, so could not answer the charges. Investigations by the sheriffs of London revealed that William had indeed died on 24 June in London, and had been buried promptly the following day in the city's Franciscan friary.[223] A charter of Edward III probably increased the risk of contamination, since from 1337 to at least 1350, it compelled merchant strangers to board with a citizen and not keep their own households or societies while in the city,[224] thus ensuring a complete mixing of residents and aliens.

Continuing fatalities among Londoners are implied elsewhere by the replacement by the king of two of his officers in June. On the 1st, Robert de Mildenhale was appointed keeper of the changes (the mint) of the Tower of London and Canterbury with the same conditions of work as his predecessor, John de Horton; and on the 8th, he granted for life to Hankin de Braban, one of his falconers, the keeping of his mews at Charing (Cross) by Westminster, 'in the same manner as John de Sancto Albano, deceased, held it'.[225] The king was also obliged to replace clergy in two further city churches, presenting John de Fakenham, chaplain, to St Matthew Friday Street on 20 June, and Simon de Brantyngham to St Alphege Cripplegate on 27 June.[226] The latter presentation was on account of the fact that the dean of St Martin-le-Grand (the religious house which normally had rights of presentation) had also died. On 19 June Edward had selected William de Cusantia, a canon of St Paul's, as the new dean,[227] but his position was yet to be confirmed.

Plague stalked the city and guilds, too. At a Court of Pleas held on 11 June, members of the woolmongers elected Peter Sterre to replace William Dyry, deceased, to the office of tronage of wools in the city and suburbs; on

24 June William Raven, mercer, was elected to the office of the Small Balance, paying 50s yearly to the chamberlain. He was to last at the most a fortnight before he too succumbed, and was replaced in his turn on 7 July by Simon de Reynham.[228]

The most significant event of the month was without doubt Edward's issue of the Ordinance of Labourers, on 18 June. The king presented a writ to every sheriff and bishop in the land, setting out a response to what he saw as an alarming rise in inflation driven by spiralling wages. A 'great part of the population has now died in this pestilence', he noted, and as a consequence, contracted workers were refusing to work unless they were paid an excessive salary. He also concluded that many 'prefer to beg in idleness rather than work for their living'. Having taken counsel from his nobles and prelates, he had ordained the following:

 − All those below 60 years, fit, having neither trade, professional craft or private lands and means, and currently unemployed, must take up employment if it is offered, but for wages at the levels they were in 1346.
 − Any proven to have refused such work should be jailed until they recant.
 − No employers should offer remuneration greater than 1346 levels, and any who do, should be tried in appropriate courts, with a forfeiture of twice or triple the offered wage to anyone adversely affected by the offer.
 − Those who have already workers on at a higher salary than 1346 levels must revert the salary on pain of penalties.
 − Reapers and mowers cannot leave their current employment before the agreed term is completed, on pain of imprisonment.
 − Saddlers, skinners, tawyers, cobblers, tailors, smiths, carpenters, masons, tilers, shipwrights, carters, and all other artisans and labourers are bound to work for 1346 wages levels.
 − Butchers, fishmongers, innkeepers, brewers, bakers, poulterers, and all other dealers in foodstuffs, are bound to sell produce at a reasonable price. Those charging higher will pay twice the sum charged in recompense, if proven (bailiffs not enforcing the ordinance will be liable to pay triple the charge if proven).
 − Beggars who are able to work should not receive alms, with contravention punishable by prison, so that they will be forced to work for a living.
 − The bishops were also to moderate the income of stipendiary chaplains many of whom it seemed were refusing to serve without an excessive salary, under pain of suspension and interdict.
 − This ordinance was to be proclaimed by sheriffs in all cities, boroughs, market towns and ports, and wherever else the sheriffs deem appropriate.

– The bishops were further exhorted to publish the ordinance in every church, and direct the clergy to exhort every parishioner to obey the ordinances. [229]

This extraordinary and draconian attempt to deny the inevitable effects of a diminished labour pool must have seemed like the ultimate punishment for a population reeling from the principal effects of the plague, and indeed still dying in considerable numbers from it. The very fact that the king considered it necessary illustrates the extent to which that labour pool must have been reduced by the plague.

July 1349

The implementation of the ordinance in London, recorded in the City Letter Books in July 1349, provides us with some indirect evidence for the passage of the plague itself: while the king's writ spoke of the population that have 'now' died in this pestilence, the Letter Book records that the ordinance is in consequence of the 'recent' pestilence. [230] The plague had been spreading into the northern parts of the country as the writ was sent out, and so was indeed current in some parts, but in London, the wording clearly signals that the plague was considered to be abating.

Almost immediately, cases were brought to court under the new ordinances. On 18 July William de Osprenge, Ralph atte Hoke, John Chaumpeneys, William de Bergeveny, John de la Maneys, Martin le Mynour of Holborn and other bakers' servants were indicted for forming a conspiracy among themselves that they would not work for their masters except at double or treble the wages formerly given. They pleaded not guilty and demanded a jury. The employers were also obviously affected by the ordinances, and the bakers asked the mayor to clarify the terms of service under which such servants as the alleged conspirators represented might be taken on. It was determined that no servant should contract for less than three months, and that wages should be paid in arrears at the end of each period, as with other guilds. A fine of 40s, payable to the city chamberlain, was appointed for any infraction of these rules. [231]

Truly this must have been a miserable time for the low-paid: their income had been capped despite the price rises permitted (so their puchasing power must have dipped dangerously), and compounding matters, they were required to cover their costs for months before any payment would come in. It can only have been bitterly unpopular, and 'occasioned greater hardships than even the pestilence, for whilst the latter made labour scarce and had conduced to higher wages, the [ordinance] offered wages to the labourer that it was worse than slavery to accept'.[232]

July brought a further drop in mortality, and in the expectation of mortality. Of the wills enrolled in Husting, only six were drawn up in the month. Significantly, of these, three were written for people who did not wish burial in a London location: Conwy, Hertfordshire and Kent were the places mentioned.[233] If these were people who simply had a particular interest in the city, but did not dwell there, then the will-making rate had effectively returned to normal levels. One notable Londoner who drew his will up was John de Gildesburgh,[234] the fishmonger who had developed Desebourne Lane near Queenhithe in the previous September. His will requested burial in his chantry chapel in the parish church of St Mary Somerset, and additionally left a bequest of 60s to the service of a charnel in the church.[235] It may be expected that the charnel functions of many parish churches had been considerably expanded as a result of the plague, given the intensive use of cemetery space required. Gildesburgh's will was enrolled in October, but since the Husting court was suspended for August and September, it is possible he died shortly after making it.

While will-making had dropped away, enrolments in July actually increased on the previous month to a total of fifty-one, up by twenty wills on the June figure. This substantial increase simply represents a lag in the presentation of the wills during the period of the Boston fair between 17 June and 16 July, so many of these, probably over half, would normally have been enrolled up to four weeks earlier.

Wills of note enrolled in July include that of Walter Bole, the master mason at Westminster Abbey, who requested burial at St Andrew Castle Baynard; Jordan Habraham, the distinctively named rector of St Mary Magdalen Fish Street; John de Toppesfeld, a goldsmith, and his mother Johanna, whose wills were enrolled within a week of each other; and John Palmer, the shipwright, and his wife Amy, whose wills were enrolled on the same day (despite the fact that John had perished some time earlier – good evidence that the plague was still at large).[236] Other deaths are implied or recorded in this month and in early August.

On 20 July the king presented William de Whiten as chaplain to St James Garlickhythe (the abbot's seat at Westminster still technically vacant), but was forced to appoint another chaplain, Roger de Stretford, just three weeks later.[237] Further royal appointments included John de Brampton, replacing the deceased Richard Yenge, to manage the supply of glass and glaziers for the chapel at Westminster Palace; and John Styrop as keeper of the king's lions at the Tower of London, replacing Robert de Doncastre, deceased.[238]

How many of these could be blamed on plague is not clear (and we have especially to wonder about the lion-keeper), but the emphasis on the deaths of officers is probably significant. It may be this obstinate refusal of the plague to die down completely that prompted King Edward to transport his varied and extensive collection of religious relics from the Tower to the palace at King's Langley (Bucks) on 4 July 1349.[239]

Mortality was certainly still in evidence in the manor of Stepney, where the court had not sat for more than two months since April. Two sessions were held: one on 6 July recorded forty-five deaths (presumably relating to May and June in the main); but another, three weeks later on 30 July, mentions a further twenty-nine deaths, suggesting that the epidemic was still at large.[240]

August 1349

The number of wills drawn up in August (three) and September (two) approached normal pre-plague levels, and the language contained in one clearly indicates that the focus of attention was the consequence of the plague for others, not personal preservation and salvation. Hugh de Robury, a wealthy glover described in his will as a 'brother' of the Augustinian houses of Holy Trinity, Aldgate and St Mary Overie, Southwark, left considerable sums to several religious houses and many of London's hospitals. The remainder he set aside to be divided among 'those who, having been reduced from affluence to poverty, are ashamed to get a livelihood by begging; and those poor men who come up from the rural districts to the City of London to get a living by selling brushwood, timber, heather and other things'.[241] This is perhaps our clearest evidence of the immediate human consequences in the city both of the plague itself and of the Ordinance of Labourers. A similarly pathetic image is conjured by the imprisonment on 20 August of John de Goldstone of Barking, John de Clayhurst and Walter Sprot of Greenwich for using 'false' nets in the Thames on the east side of London Bridge, to catch 'three bushels of small fish ... which fish, by reason of their smallness, could be of no use to any one'.[242] Such economic distress is evident from north of the city in Hertfordshire as early as August, where some refused to pay their taxes; resisting collectors by force of arms and by appropriating the assets of the plague dead. The king's response was uncompromising, threatening prison to all defaulters.[243]

Another immediate consequence of the fading of the plague's virulence was the increase in the number of guardianships of orphaned children being ratified in the mayor's court. Goldsmith Richard de Basyngstoke had died of plague in early May. At the end of July his son, aged just 1½ years, was committed to the care of John de Depleye and his wife Johanna, described as the child's mother: Johanna, having lost her husband, had evidently remarried within two months,[244] a situation that may well have been repeated frequently throughout the city. The effect of this coping strategy on the social network in the city must have been profound.

Trade networks also played a significant part in redistributing the responsibilities of care for orphans of wealthier citizens. Roger Syward, a pewterer, made a will on 30 October 1348 (enrolled on 20 July 1349) which mentioned a wife and six children. Roger, his wife and three of the children were dead by August, when guardianship of the surviving offspring – William, 6, Mary, 5, and Thomas, aged 1½ years – was committed to John Syward, also a pewterer. The necessary sureties to underpin the commitment were offered by three other pewterers, undoubtedly members of the craft guild.[245] Such mechanisms for social care of the wealthier families serve also to remind us how very vulnerable the surviving poor of the city must have been – there is no written evidence for the strategies they employed, but it has to be assumed that the weakest members of society, those children, disabled and elderly who had lost their principal supporting family, must have been in very dire straits.

The guardianship strategy itself did not always work well; economic exigencies and human greed combined to tempt at least some guardians into keeping for themselves goods and estates that had been entrusted to children of plague victims. In September such cases began to come before the mayor and aldermen. On 7 September Robert de Wodham, executor of the original executor of one John le Parmenter, was summoned to answer a complaint from le Parmenter's close friends, William Spershore and his wife Joan. Spershore claimed that Wodham was withholding goods meant for the children of le Parmenter. In court he agreed he was holding '£30, a signet ring and other goods and chattels' for them. He was made to pay 27s 2d for the goods and the £30 in gold nobles to the city chamberlain, who in turn paid it to Spershore for Elena, the sole surviving child. This transfer of guardianship to the friends of the family was formalised in a later court in December.[246]

Goods and money were also at risk of theft until a formal handover could take place. On 26 August 1349 friends of a dead draper, John de Sellyng, came to plead at court that John de Cantebrigge, a chaplain, was withholding from Sellyng's daughters, Margery and Juliana, £10 left to them by their father. The money had been passed to Sellyng's executor, Henry de Asshebourn, and on his death into the hands of his executor, de Cantebrigge.

The latter pleaded that he had duly administered de Asshebourn's estate and only 5 marks were left. However, the jury found that he still had in his possession sufficient goods belonging to the testator to pay the £10 due to the children, and judgement was given that he pay up. On 2 September, Chaplain John de Pampesworth and Amy de Rokesbourgh came to court. They were further executors of Henry de Asshebourn and accused two men, Robert de Hyngeston and Simon de Chikesond, of stealing 'a sack of wool, 13 silver spoons, and silver rings, buckles and cups, belonging to the children of the said John de Sellyng'. The jury found for the plaintiffs and the defendants were imprisoned. Two weeks later the court received the £10 from John de Cantebrigge.[247]

It was not just the goods and money that were at risk in this turbulent time – the orphans themselves might be abducted. The will of John de Leche, ironmonger, left his daughter Alice in the guardianship of his wife Matilda. It also made provision for a chantry in St Michael Cornhill, and for pious uses for the souls of his family and of a friend, Thomas de Northerne, who had died in January 1349. De Leche died before 2 March, the date of probate. However, over seven years later, in May 1356, a case was brought before the mayor and aldermen by the rector of St Michael's, reporting that de Leche's wife had died in mid-Lent 1349 (less than three weeks after her husband), and Stephen de Northerne, Thomas' brother, had assumed guardianship of Alice, de Leche's now-orphaned daughter. The rector alleged that Stephen 'had seized and wasted the property of the said Alice, to the prejudice of certain chantries, and had eloigned the said Alice, aged eight years, out of the City'.[248]

The transfer of goods and bequests could be highly complex, even when no guardians were involved, due simply to the rate of death among beneficiaries. In March 1349 Peter Nayere, an armourer, bequeathed to Nicholas Blake, his son, £88 6s 8d for the support of Blake's four sisters. Blake, who died before 31 October 1349, in turn left the money in trust to John de Gildeforde. De Gildeforde also died before the end of November, leaving the money to his own executors, who in turn presented the money to the chamberlain of the city in trust. On 1 December three surviving Blake sisters claimed the money from the chamberlain.[249]

It is difficult to estimate how many Londoners actually died in August and September, for these were closed months as far as the Husting was concerned, allowing for the management of harvest and attendance at fairs; no wills for this period were therefore enrolled. However, some key individuals certainly did perish in the city, and probably of the plague. Most notable was the Archbishop-elect of Canterbury, Thomas Bradwardine. Following his election to replace John de Offord in July 1349, he 'hurried to London, but died [on 26 August 1349] in the hostel of the Bishop of Rochester at La Place [near Lambeth] where he had lain sick for four days'.[250] He was replaced immediately by Simon Islip, who was consecrated unusually at St Paul's not Canterbury, much to the discontent of the monks at the latter seat. One month later, on 30 September, John Shenche, the keeper of Westminster Palace and the Fleet prison, also died.[251] The fear of further mortality at Westminster Abbey must surely be the reason why no fewer than seven senior monks there, including the abbot, infirmarer, precentor and cellarer, nearly one-third of the surviving convent, all sought, and on 11 August received, papal dispensation to seek their own confessors.[252] So the plague lurked throughout the summer, but there appears to be no basis for the assertion made by some that the period between June and September was the most virulent.[253]

The fact that the plague had not yet died out may also explain a remarkable event reported by the eye-witness Robert of Avesbury. Around Michaelmas, he reported:

> more than 120 men, for the most part from Zeeland or Holland, arrived in London from Flanders. They went barefoot in procession twice a day in the sight of the people, sometimes in St Paul's church, sometimes elsewhere in the city, their bodies naked except for a linen cloth from loins to ankle. Each wore a hood painted with a red cross at front and back and carried in his right hand a whip with three thongs.[254]

These were the Flagellants, religious zealots who scourged themselves in reparation for the sins of the world, and who had appeared as a movement nearly a century before. They had emerged as early as 1348 in response to the arrival of pestilence in mainland Europe, and had again attracted the disfavour of the Pope who saw in them a threat to the stability of the Church. Evidently, the perceived threat from these religious fanatics continued to manifest itself at least until the end of the year, for in October and again in December, the Pope felt compelled to write to the king: 'on the superstitious and vain society [of Flagellants] in Almain and elsewhere, against whom a papal constitution has been sent to all prelates, a copy of which is enclosed, and requesting the king, should any of them enter his kingdom, to drive them out of it'.[255]

The Plague Withers

Naturally, a backlog of will enrolments was created by the two-month hiatus in the Husting court of August and September,[256] and we must jump to the months of October and November to see the level of mortality occurring among the richer classes across later summer and autumn. In total, eighteen wills were enrolled in October, increasing to twenty-seven in November. Taking all four months into account, there was clearly a downward trend, averaging out at about ten enrolments per month – a very considerable drop from the July figure. Furthermore, in October four of the eighteen wills related to those wishing burial away from London.

Nonetheless, mortality was still elevated, each month accounting for half of a normal year's enrolment. Several wills of note appear in the rolls. That of the great merchant and financier, and four times mayor of the city, John de Pulteney (d. 6 June 1349), was proved on 19 October; he wished to be buried in St Paul's Cathedral and left among his great estate his mansion called Coldharbour, valued at £1,000. Family tragedies continued to strike, with the wills of William Haunsard made in August, and of his son, also called William, dated in October, both being enrolled on the same day, 9 November.

Families also made attempts to be rejoined in death: Richard de Monoye, a cook, wished burial in a tomb in the church of St Thomas Acon beside the bones of his son; Johanna Werlyngworth near those of her husband in the churchyard of St Paul's; William Passefeld near his wife in the same cemetery; and William de Bernes at the head of his father's tomb in St Peter-the-Less. De Bernes, a fishmonger whose will was enrolled on 26 October, left his three children in the guardianship of another fishmonger, William de Hedrisham. However, he too was dead within two weeks and the children found themselves transferred into the care of the chaplain of St Peter-the-Less.[257] This strongly suggests the continuing menace of the plague.

Other, less spiritual matters were in the minds of some testators. Gilbert le Palmer's will left, among other things, money to repair the principal highways within 20 miles of the city, and it would appear that they were in some need of attention, since on 4 December the king issued a commission to determine who should repair 'many bridges on the highways between the city of London and Croydon and Kyngeston, and other places' described as 'broken down and dangerous'.[258] Whether this was as a result of neglect during the plague, or a more general campaign to restore the communication and transport infrastructure, is unclear.

Infrastructure of a different sort was being addressed within the guilds. The plague had carried off many elected representatives and attempts are visible to restore order and management. In November 1349 an election was held to replace the nine wardens of the cutlers' guild named in 1344. It is noteworthy that only six new wardens are named – either the need for, or the availability of, suitable candidates had diminished by one-third.[259]

The impact of the mortality on Husting court business can be gauged by a report from sheriffs that twelve out of sixteen witnesses to one particular deed had died in the pestilence.[260] The hearing of Possessory Assizes began again on 7 November, and began to deal with cases arising from property disputes during the plague.[261] One case gives us a taste of the dislocation created by the disaster at first hand. William de Newenham had complained that in April 1347 he had been dispossessed of a shop in the parish of St Gregory, near the cathedral, by three men – a tailor, a baker and a plasterer. The case was suspended first in July 1347 since no jury could be assembled, and then three more times during the summer of 1348 at the agreement of both parties. The case was reviewed in November 1349 and a fine issued to de Newenham for not prosecuting his case; but the unfortunate plaintiff was beyond caring – he had perished of the plague at least six months earlier.[262]

December 1349 saw deaths and will-making both at a level that was almost normal for pre-plague years. Just seven wills were enrolled, including those of the wives of two bell-founders (termed 'potters' in the documents). Agnes de Romeneye was the wife of bell-founder John, who had died in April 1349.[263] Matilda was the wife of Peter de Weston and mother of Thomas, both of whom were significant bell-founders. Peter had died before the plague in 1347; Thomas succumbed in April 1349. Remarkably, several of their bells still ring across the English countryside, cast by Peter at Tattenhoe in Buckinghamshire (*c.* 1330); Bethersden in Kent (*c.* 1335); Whitwell on the Isle of Wight; Kingsbury in Middlesex (*c.* 1347); and Thomas at Chalk in Kent. The inscription on this bell reads '*xpe: pie: flos: marie*', urging the Blessed Virgin's mercy to flow from its ringing. It is noteworthy that the annals of Dunstable priory record that in the year of the plague the townspeople made themselves a bell and called it Maria.[264] While many bells were doubtless given this name, the Virgin's intercessory powers against God's wrath carried great weight and it might well be one example of a spiritual response to the plague.

The Ordinance of Labourers continued to cause trouble among London workers, and on 21 November, and again on 8 December, the king felt compelled to issue another writ to the mayor and sheriffs to forbid 'artificers and others' demanding higher wages than before the pestilence, on pain of imprisonment.[265] Examples are frequent in the Pleas and Memoranda rolls of continued attempts to subvert this hugely unpopular edict over the second half of 1349. In September, two bakers in St Botolph's Lane pleaded guilty to the charge of paying their men part of their wages during the quarter (rather than at the end), contrary to the ordinance. In October, butchers were sworn to see that their colleagues did not charge more for meat than was customary before the plague; a considerable number of wine-sellers were thrown temporarily into Newgate gaol for charging double the appropriate sums for their wares; and leather-sellers and shoemakers were prosecuted for over-pricing their goods. In November, William Amery, mason, was imprisoned for refusing to do work valued at 12*d* at St Christopher's church for less than 5*s*, and a 'conspiracy' of over sixty cordwainers' servants to fix wage levels was unmasked – an early experiment at unionisation perhaps.[266]

The economic upheaval created by the plague appears to have led to much wider population movements. On 1 December the king issued a writ to the mayor and sheriffs of London that they proclaim none should leave the kingdom 'except well-known merchants, inasmuch as the country had become so much depopulated by the pestilence and the Treasury exhausted'.[267] The city itself appears to have become a magnet for migrants, 'a great concourse of aliens and denizens', many armed and seemingly oblivious of any curfew. City authorities were already making arrests when, on 29 December, Edward placed full royal support behind those attempting to keep the king's peace, demanding punishment of all transgressors, 'now that the pestilence is stayed'.[268] What part the Ordinance of Labourers might have played in any civil unrest at this time is unclear, but it cannot have helped matters as surviving families and businesses tried to return to something like a normal footing. Confirmation that the plague had run its course, at least in the south of the country, came from a letter written by Simon Islip, Archbishop of Canterbury, on 28 December to the Bishop of London. In it, urging public expressions of gratitude to God, he recalled 'the amazing pestilence which lately attacked these parts and which took from us by far the best and worthiest men'.[269]

Just three wills were drawn up and four wills enrolled in Husting during January 1350, apparently confirming the conclusion of the pestilence. However, there is circumstantial evidence that either late in that month, or in February, the city was visited with either a fresh outbreak or an entirely different disease, something which lasted through March and into April or even May. The evidence shows up in the Husting wills for spring: while there was no change in the number of wills drawn up (zero in February, three in March and two in April), a spike of seventeen were enrolled in February, falling to eight in March and six in April. Of the wills enrolled in February, those of John Miles of Hosier Lane in West Smithfield, and his wife Matilda, were both enrolled on the same day;[270] while the will of Alice de Hakeneye, wife of Richard, a former alderman, was proved on the same day that her son Richard was confirmed legal guardian of his little sister, Isabella.[271] Both examples provide plausible indicators of sudden death.

The increase in rates of enrolment appears to coincide with a curious hiatus in the account rolls for construction work at the Tower of London.[272] Between February and May 1350 almost no wages were paid out to the crews who were working right through the plague months, and who, from June onwards, resumed work at very nearly pre-plague levels (over £14 per month until September). The roll on which these blank months show up is complete, and work certainly was not finished. It is conceivable that the workers were moved to a different royal construction project, though there is no evidence for this; it may therefore be more likely that the labourers, along with a number of other Londoners, were affected by disease.

Matters were clearly also worrying the city authorities at this time, since before February they attempted to ensure that blanket absolution for the city was available. One Nicholas de Hethe (then a canon of St Paul's, Salisbury and Hereford[273]), recommended by John Worthin, a Dominican friar in London, having exceptional influence with the Pope, had taken more than £40 from former mayor Andrew Aubrey with which to procure bulls of absolution for the whole city. De Hethe had subsequently confirmed that the bulls had been purchased, but by 6 February there was no sign of them. The mayor thus wrote, stating plainly that unless the bulls appeared, de Hethe would be prosecuted and the Pope made fully aware of his deception.[274] It is clear that de Hethe could not produce the bulls, for on 2 April 1350 the mayor petitioned the Pope directly to request that the friar, John Worthin, be given the power of absolution that the bulls were intended to furnish. In rich language, the letter explained that:

> a dreadful mortality has so cut off our merchants, that our citizens who … are no longer able in person to visit your most Holy See, even though they should be involved in cases which are reserved for your Court, without a ruinous expense, while the present wars are going on. With one accord therefore, with weeping does your congregation here entreat the most exalted highness of your Holiness, that the same your Holiness will deign graciously to grant unto the venerable and religious man, Brother John de Worthyn, your Chaplain, a man of honour, of approved life, manners, and learning, sprung from the high blood of our realm, who alone, of all others, strengthens us with the word of Christ … that he, and he only within our city, may be able to absolve our people, being penitent; and to enjoin salutary penances upon them according to the nature of their fault.

The letter further requested that in the event of Worthin's death, another Dominican friar might be appointed in his place.[275]

The development of the East Smithfield emergency cemetery took a fresh turn in March 1350. John Cory, the clerk who had been acquiring lands around the site of the cemetery since before the plague, granted to the king 'all his messuages at Tourhulle adjoining the new churchyard of Holy Trinity by the Tower of London'. This was no small land transaction: its witnesses included the Chancellor of England, the treasurer, the king's chamberlain and two knights. Two days later, on 20 March, Edward granted the land on to the 'president and monks of the house of the Cistercian order, to be called the royal free chapel of St Mary Graces', which he had decided to found and endow 'in the new graveyard of the Holy Trinity by the Tower of London'.[276] A new Cistercian abbey was in the making in the shadow of the Tower, and its proposed site was the plague cemetery. Edward's motivation for founding an abbey was complex, but the establishment of a permanent memorial to his late confessor, Thomas Bradwardine, the Archbishop of Canterbury who had died in Lambeth of the pestilence, may have been one catalyst and may have influenced his choice of location.[277] Within a year, Walter de Mauny would consider an enlargement of the college of priests in the West Smithfield plague cemetery. Just how wise the monks and priests thought these plans were is not recorded, but the founding of two new religious houses in immediate proximity to the plague dead marks a clear reconciliation process: the emergency was over and the spiritual reconfiguration of the mass burial sites was under way.

By April 1350, therefore, the immediate events connected with the first, greatest outbreak of the pestilence had concluded. The core of the epidemic had lasted in the city for nine months from November through to the end of July, with an intermittently spiking level of mortality from then until March 1350. The survivors and the newcomers faced a very different city to that of eighteen months earlier.

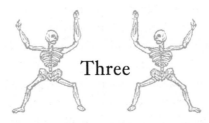

Three

THE GREAT MORTALITY

LONDON SUFFERED the plague for nine months, from the beginning of November 1348 to the end of July 1349, with some less convincing evidence of spikes of mortality through to March 1350. The evidence presented provides a monthly snapshot of the developing plague, but an overview of the anatomy of the disaster is also to some extent possible. This chapter examines the speed of spread, the impact on administration, the evidence for dealing with the dead, the final death toll, and some immediate impacts on the survivors.

Coping with the Pestilence

The way in which the city and its residents were able to cope, as a body rather than individually, was dependent on the speed and scale of the disaster. Fig. 6 shows the rate at which Husting wills were drawn up compared with the rate of their subsequent enrolment. It includes the monthly averages of reported deaths from the adjacent manor of Stepney.

The early November start date is confirmed by an increase in mortality and will-making at precisely this time. Monthly death rates indicated by the Stepney evidence track the will-making curve very closely, suggesting that the latter may accurately represent the mortality curve for the city. The known dates for the founding of the three emergency cemeteries – December for Stratford's Pardon churchyard, January for Walter de Mauny's

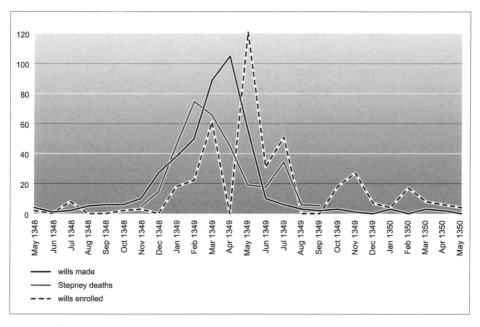

Fig. 6 Wills made, and enrolled, in the Husting court, May 1348 to May 1350, and deaths notified in the Bishop of London's manor court at Stepney between November 1348 and September 1349. (Sources: Calendar of Husting Wills; TNA SC 2/191/60)

Newchirchehaw, and probably February for the Cemetery of the Holy Trinity near the Tower – fit this accelerating death curve perfectly. The speed with which the plague spread and infected the citizens was undoubtedly greater than is implied by the evidence of the will enrolments, the curve of which lags considerably behind both of the others. This can be tested using a sample of cases where additional evidence for the date of death is available from supplementary sources.

For eighteen wills made during the plague months, the date of death can be narrowed down to a *terminus ante quem*, lying between the date the will was drawn up and that of its enrolment (see Table 1). In several instances the exact day of death is known. The sources which provide us with this information most frequently are the subsequent wills of family members drawn up after the deaths of the individual concerned, but before enrolment; but others include chance references to obits or court cases regarding estates brought by survivors.

The sample (4.6 per cent) is small, but it suggests that the period between will-making and probate was just under one-quarter (23.7 per cent) of the period between will-making and enrolment.[278] If true, of the 392 wills made in the plague months, 60 per cent of the will-makers would have died within

SURNAME	W = WILL MADE	D = DEATH BY/ON	EH = ENROLLED IN HUSTING	W TO D IN DAYS	D TO EH IN DAYS	TOTAL DAYS	% W–D	% D–EH
Hamond, J.	02-Oct-48	20-Oct-48	09-Feb-49	18	112	130	13.8	86.2
Pulteney, J.	14-Nov-48	06-Jun-49	19-Oct-49	206	126	332	62	38
Hicchen, J.	28-Nov-48	02-Dec-48	02-Mar-49	4	91	95	4.2	95.8
Neve, J.	18-Dec-48	08-Apr-49	04-May-49	99	26	125	79.2	20.8
Sampford, J.	20-Dec-48	01-Jan-49	20-Jan-49	12	19	31	38.7	61.3
Hemenhale, E.	26-Dec-48	13-Jan-49	19-Oct-49	19	282	301	6.3	93.7
Hanhampsted, W.	02-Jan-49	29-May-49	20-Jul-49	146	52	198	73.7	26.3
Fraunceys, T.	13-Feb-49	14-Feb-49	23-Mar-49	1	37	38	2.6	97.4
Warefeld, J.	13-Mar-49	17-Apr-49	04-May-49	42	17	59	71.2	28.8
Mymmes, R.	14-Mar-49	23-Mar-49	30-May-51	9	796	805	1.1	98.9
Mymmes, J.	19-Mar-49	10-Apr-49	04-May-49	22	24	46	47.8	52.2
Larmurer, N.	21-Mar-49	22-Mar-49	23-Mar-49	1	1	2	50	50
Elsing, W.	23-Mar-49	03-Apr-49	04-May-49	12	32	44	27.3	72.7
Shordych, R.	26-Mar-49	05-Apr-49	25-May-49	10	50	60	16.7	83.3
Dallynge, J. Snr	06-Apr-49	20-May-49	16-Nov-49	44	175	219	20.1	79.9
Maryns, T.	22-Apr-49	25-Apr-49	11-May-49	3	16	19	15.8	84.2
Wychingham, G.	30-Apr-49	15-May-49	08-Jun-49	15	24	39	38.5	61.5
Werlyngworth, N.	01-May-49	05-May-49	19-Jul-49	4	74	78	5.1	94.9
			median	13.5	43.5		23.7	76.3

Table 1. Husting will-makers whose dates of death are known. Bold entries indicate exact dates of death; others are dates by which we know the individual had died.

twenty-one days of making their wills, and 20 per cent within five days. This suggests that death took place much closer to the date that the will was drawn up than the Husting enrolments imply. Using only the seven (1.8 per cent) individuals whose exact death dates are known, these figures would be even higher, at 33.7 per cent of will-makers dead within five days, and 68.1 per cent within three weeks. The chroniclers' tales of few surviving beyond five days appears to be supported. Using this crude model of likely death date for all 392 wills, the mortality rate for the city reached its peak in early April, probably around Easter time (which fell on the 12th that year), and about six weeks later than the Stepney manor vills. The plague had come to the city at the beginning of winter and had peaked by early spring.

There are no documents which establish the day-to-day experiences of Londoners as the plague took hold. How the city coped is visible only in its administrative accounts, contained in the Letter Books and court proceedings. It is clear that the administrative structures of the city remained functioning throughout the entire outbreak, and that the mayor, aldermen and other officials continued to conduct business as required. A summary analysis (see Table 2) of the evidence indicates that on average, officials met in some capacity almost five times each month, with a barely perceptible reduction in frequency in January and February 1349. Administrative work focused on the enrolment of wills and deeds relating to property but also covered such matters as guardianship, the swearing-in of officials and guild representatives, and, from July 1349, the prosecution of cases arising from the Ordinance of Labourers. The single longest break in the year was for twenty-five days from late March to late April which, while it coincided

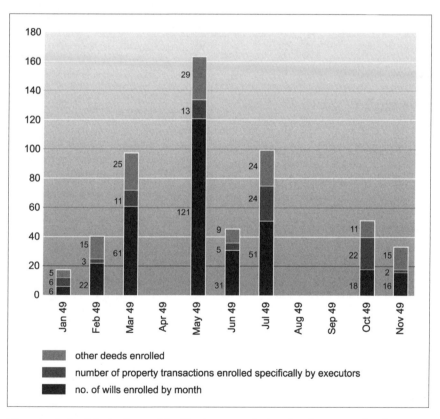

Fig. 7 Analysis of the business of the Husting court during the plague months of 1349. (Source: CHW, LMA microfiche X109/426: Wills = no of wills enrolled by month; Exec = number of property transactions enrolled specifically by executors; Other = other deeds enrolled)

	NO OF MEETINGS	DATE RANGE	BUSINESS COVERED
November 1348	6	10th–27th	Wills, Common Pleas, Pleas of Land, sureties for children, swearing-in of Sheathers' and Weavers' bailiffs
December 1348	3	5th–22nd	Guardianship case; two property assignments
January 1349	3	13th–26th	Wills, Common Pleas, Pleas of Land, two property assignments
February 1349	3	3rd–16th	Wills, Common Pleas (x 2), Pleas of Land
March 1349	7	2nd–26th	Wills, Common Pleas (x 2), Pleas of Land (x 2), false imprisonment case, demise of Bailiff of Southwark, swearing-in of Serjeant of Chamber, guardianship case
April 1349	2	20th–22nd	Swearing-in of Serjeant of Chamber, guardianship case
May 1349	6	4th–29th	Wills, Common Pleas (x 2), Pleas of Land, witness money for apprenticeship, enquiry into unpaid debt, election of Chamberlain, enquiry into boundary dispute
June 1349	3	8th–17th	Wills, Common Pleas, election of officer of tronage of wool, enquiry into unpaid debt
July 1349	7	1st–30th	Wills, Common Pleas, Pleas of Land, swearing-in of officer of Small Balance, indictment for wages conspiracy, election of brokers and measures of woad, two guardianship cases
August 1349	3	13th–26th	Certification of salt measure and carriage, guardianship case, suit over money held for minors
September 1349	6	1st–18th	Case contravening Ordinance of Labourers, plaint of intrusion into property, Assize of Nuisance on property, acknowledgement of money for guardianship, theft/withholding of minors' bequest (x 2), charge of illegal fishnets
October 1349	6	3rd–26th	Wills, Common Pleas, Pleas of Land, receipt of ex-Chamberlain's account, proclamation of king's alnager of cloth and deputy, Butchers on oath to sell at correct prices, charges of breaking Ordinance of Labourers against Winedrawers and Cordwainers, charge of overpricing against Curriers

Table 2. Summary of the frequency of civic administrative business recorded during the first outbreak. (Source: CLB, CAN, CPMR, CHW, Husting Deeds). It is not always clear how many aldermen and other officials attended the meetings, but each one mentioned above had at least two officials in attendance.

with the highest rate of will-making, was probably more to do with the normal break in sessions for Pleas than the effects of the pestilence.

The (almost) regular weekly sessions for Common Pleas and Pleas of Land dealt with the enrolment of all the deeds and wills in the Husting court; the number of enrolments and their purpose provide a snapshot of the changing nature of the business from month to month (see Fig. 7).[279]

This summary shows the proportions and numbers of enrolments relating to wills, property deeds enrolled specifically by executors of those who had died, and other enrolments concerning property. Several points are clear. First, the increasing number of wills being enrolled as a result of the plague is very obvious (April, August and September were traditionally free of sessions), but there is no consequent reduction in enrolling other deeds. It must be assumed that the sessions sat for longer to conduct the business. Second, the enrolments of deeds (as opposed to wills), and particularly those not apparently associated with the execution of bequests, demonstrate that

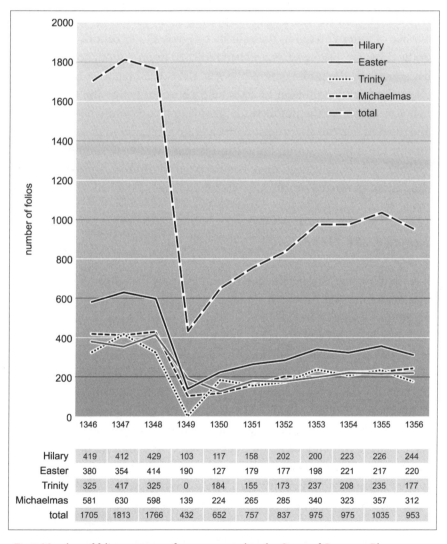

	1346	1347	1348	1349	1350	1351	1352	1353	1354	1355	1356
Hilary	419	412	429	103	117	158	202	200	223	226	244
Easter	380	354	414	190	127	179	177	198	221	217	220
Trinity	325	417	325	0	184	155	173	237	208	235	177
Michaelmas	581	630	598	139	224	265	285	340	323	357	312
total	1705	1813	1766	432	652	757	837	975	975	1035	953

Fig. 8 Number of folios per term of cases presented to the Court of Common Pleas, Westminster. (Source: TNA CP/40, provided by Graham Dawson)

property transfer continued unabated during the plague. Third, executors came in increased numbers in July and October 1349, a point which supports a general belief that the plague had slowed by July.

National judicial apparatus also had a base close to London. The Court of the Common Pleas (the Common Bench) was based at Westminster Hall and the sessions generated a number of rolls during the year.[280] These were ordered in four terms (Hilary, Easter, Trinity and Michaelmas), in which sessions were conducted, and so the crude level of business of the courts can be established by examining the trends in the number of folios for each term in each year. The folios and the numbers for 1346–53 are set out in Fig. 8. Even allowing for the immediate disruptions to die off in 1349 and 1350, the number of folios entered in the rolls in 1351 was 43 per cent of the average for the three pre-plague years, and had returned to only about 60 per cent of that average by the mid-1350s. While it is clear that a range of factors must have influenced the number of cases being brought before the Bench (and each year after 1349 the numbers are gradually rising), and while it must be remembered that the court dealt with cases from all around the country and not just London, the strong impression is that there were simply far fewer plaintiffs or defendants than there had been before. And so civic and national administration carried on: the city was by no means paralysed.

Burying the Dead

As with the living, no specific description exists of the range of people who died or the manner in which London managed the burial of its dead, but we do have tangible archaeological evidence from which to draw. For the Pardon churchyard and Newchurchehawe cemeteries this is currently limited to traces of burials: in the former, a group of five undated and disturbed burials near Great Sutton Street, and in the latter, a single burial of probable fourteenth-century date within Charterhouse Square, and a possible medieval burial on Glasshouse Yard.[281] However, for the east cemetery of the Holy Trinity we have much better evidence. In 1986 a major excavation conducted by the Museum of London revealed a very significant portion of the East Smithfield cemetery founded by those unknown 'substantial men' of the city in January or February 1349. The excavation revealed no fewer than 787 burials that could be directly linked to the 1349 outbreak, along with a number of later burials, some of which were related to Edward's abbey and some of which, it will be argued, were related to later outbreaks of pestilence in the fourteenth century. It remains, worldwide, the only major excavation of an emergency cemetery which was set up during this first (and greatest) outbreak. It provides our only window on the city's numerous poor, those largely invisible in the story set out in Chapter 2, and sheds important light on the manner in which London's emergency cemeteries were conceived and operated.

The cemetery of the Holy Trinity lay immediately east of the city wall adjacent to the Tower of London. It was bounded on the north by Hog Street (Hoggestrete), now Royal Mint Street, and on the south by East Smithfield. Two specific areas were set out in this cemetery for burial (see Fig. 4). The western area was rectangular and measured 76m by about 35m. At a distance of some 40m to the east, a second plot consisted of a long, narrow area measuring at least 125m by 12m. The third component of the cemetery was its chapel, a building now known to have been constructed as early as April 1349. A small fragment of a chalk wall foundation was located south of the western burial plot; its later association with the earliest cloister of the Cistercian abbey of St Mary Graces makes it highly likely that this was part of that chapel, reused as the first, temporary abbey chapel. If so, the cemetery chapel stood in the south-west corner of the cemetery, about 20m south of the western burial plot and 45m west of the eastern plot. In total, then, the cemetery as used comprised an area about 132m by 82m (approximately 2⅔ acres). This sits adequately within the larger footprint defined in the Cartulary of Holy Trinity priory, which had an area of about 170m by 107m. The cemetery was surrounded by an earthen wall, of which no archaeological trace was found, and was provided with a gatehouse at some point before 1359,[282] which opened westward on to Tower Hill itself.

The archaeological evidence that this cemetery provides is very rich. It allows us to consider three key issues in some detail. Firstly, the state of the corpses (whether there was evidence for clothing or a wooden coffin, for example) imparts considerable information about how families and communities prepared the victims for burial before transport to the cemetery. Second, the disposition and character of the graves and mass trenches tell us how the cemetery itself may have been managed. Third, the frequency of burial, and the demographic information revealed through the study of the skeletons themselves, provides us with a novel means of looking at the kinds of people who became victims, and a way of considering the rate at which they died.

The most helpful place to begin the archaeological enquiry is with some general facts and figures about the nature of the people buried. Altogether, the skeletons of 787 men, women and children were excavated from the first, 1349, phase of the cemetery. Of 636 of these, some aspect of the age, sex, or both, could be determined by osteoarchaeological inspection.[283] In the remainder of cases, the bone did not survive sufficiently well for study or identification, having been degraded by industrial waste leached from the later Royal Mint works.

Almost 34 per cent (216) of those buried there died before they had reached maturity (before the age of around 16), and we cannot tell their sex from the bones. Of these, a third were infants (below 5 years) and two-thirds children or teenagers. Of the 420 adults, ninety-seven could only be described as adult. The remaining 323 could be grouped into those whose sex we can determine, whose age we can determine, or both. A total of 290 adults were sufficiently well preserved to allow us to establish their sex: 65 per cent were male and 35 per cent female (a ratio of 1.86:1). Of 298 skeletons whose age could be estimated, 22 per cent were young adults (under 26 years); 71 per cent were mature (up to 45 years); and just 7 per cent were considered elderly. Age and sex could be estimated for a group of 268 adults (see Table 3a). If this pattern could be extrapolated for all 420 adult skeletons, and combined with the evidence we have for the 216 infants, children and teenagers, we might attempt a generalised guess at the original age and sex distribution of those buried in the cemetery (see Table 3b).

The difficulties presented in interpretation both of age and sex of individual skeletons emerge when the comparison of separate research programmes is made. Table 3c shows the results of another examination of a sample of 490 skeletons from the East Smithfield cemetery. It is clear that this researcher identified a greater number of children, young adults and older adults present at the expense of the number of mature adults.[284] Overall, in this interpretation nearly 40 per cent of the victims were below the age of around 16 years, a significant increase, and the contrast in the male to female ratio is less (1.34:1). Despite the inherent difficulty in arriving at hard facts about the victims which these divergent researches show, we can be reasonably sure that about 35 per cent of the dead were children and roughly half were under 25 years old; and also that more men than women were buried at this cemetery.

The total of 787 burials probably represents about one-third of all those that might originally have taken place in the cemetery, allowing for the destruction of other burials by later development and areas not available for excavation; the original figure has been estimated at some 2,400.[285] Assuming the cemetery functioned in its first phase from the end of January 1349 for six months, this would suggest that an average of about thirteen burials were made daily here, although the preceding chapter has clearly demonstrated a very high peak of mortality in March and April, and a probable lessening from

Young men (16–25 yrs)	13%	Young women	6%
Mature men (26–45 yrs)	48%	Mature women	26%
Old men (46 yrs +)	4%	Old women	6%

Table 3a. Analysis of the age and sex distribution of 265 adults from the East Smithfield cemetery (site code MIN86, data derived from Grainger et al. 2008, 26).

Infants (0–5 yrs)	10%		
Children/teens (6–15 yrs)	24%		
Young men (16–25 yrs)	9%	Young women	4%
Mature men (26–45 yrs)	31%	Mature women	16%
Old men (46 yrs +)	3%	Old women	3%

Table 3b. Reconstructed distribution of age/sex of victims from the East Smithfield cemetery, 1349.

Infants	11%		
Children/teens	28%		
Young men	12%	Young women	11%
Mature men	16%	Mature women	10%
Old men	7%	Old women	5%

Table 3c. Reconstructed distribution of age/sex of victims from the East Smithfield cemetery, 1349. (Source: sample of 490 skeletons analysed by S. DeWitte)

the end of May onwards. On that basis (and accepting we may be building surmise on supposition), we might suggest perhaps twenty to thirty burials a day for February to April, and commensurately less subsequently. While still a high figure, this is a fraction of the rate of 200 burials per day recorded by Robert of Avesbury for the much larger West Smithfield cemetery.

The physical remains of the people who were buried at East Smithfield give us a unique insight into the impact of the pestilence on the population of the city and nearby settlements. Who those buried in the cemetery were, and where they came from, is unknown. The adults were, in the main, between the ages of 25 and 45, and while any precise calculation of age at death is now impossible, the average age was probably 30–35 years. This is not dissimilar to the average age at death for the period 1413–1507 calculated for those monks of Christchurch Canterbury whose cause of death was recorded as plague.[286] The stature of the dead would seem to indicate that the group as a whole had been subjected to environmental stress during life. The height of some ninety adults (sixty men and thirty women) could be calculated: 1.68m (5ft 6in) for the men and 1.57m (5ft 2in) for the women; they were generally shorter than those of at least twelve other English later medieval cemetery assemblages.[287] This would seem to suggest that they were from the poorer segment of society.

The second clear indication from the cemetery figures is that more than one-third of the burials were of sub-adults. The number of children living in London at the outbreak of the epidemic is unknown, but this shows that, as with later plagues, the toll among the young was significant, and apparently evenly spread among infants, children and teenagers, though of course we do not know if there was a sex bias here. Certain families were clearly hit hard, such as that of William Robury, brother to the Hugh who had left funding for those brought to destitution by the plague. In 1353 a wardship hearing before the mayor and aldermen heard 'evidence having been brought showing that the said William and all his children except one, viz, Robert, aged thirteen, were dead'.[288] The pathetic sight of hundreds of small, shrouded forms being carried to the cemeteries would certainly have been sufficient to create the perception among chroniclers that the plague struck the young especially hard.

Perhaps the most intriguing aspect is the apparent mismatch between the numbers of men and women buried. This might be for a number of reasons, some technical and some cultural. The method of establishing the sex of ancient skeletons is not secure, and a bias in identification away from women and towards men is probably present. It has been proposed that as a result of the dangers of pregnancy and birth, a slight predominance of males may have existed in pre-industrial societies until the average age of female menopause, reflected in an overall greater number of men at any one time.[289] The cemetery, like West Smithfield, may have been used to bury strangers and travellers to the city and it is perhaps likely (although by no means certain at such a crisis time) that such travellers (such as traders) were rather more likely to be male: a male bias might have been introduced in this way. All of these factors may serve to drive up the proportion of males to females. However, there may be a more significant reason.

The disease itself might have struck males harder than females for some reason. As we will see, later outbreaks of pestilence were clearly reported by chroniclers to affect children and young men more than women, and a modern analysis of nearly 3,000 parish records of St Botolph Bishopsgate, relating to the epidemics of 1603 and 1625 in London, revealed that males outnumbered females between the ages of 15 and 44 by a ratio of 2:1.[290] However, such evidence as exists for the fourteenth century is not at all clear-cut. A study of the 1349 pestilence in twenty-eight townships in County Durham revealed that of a total of 718 identified tenants, 362 (almost exactly 50 per cent) died in 1349. Of the total, 155 (22 per cent) were women, and of these eighty-one (52 per cent) died, suggesting that the plague was an even-handed killer.[291] The burial register for the Dominican friary in Siena demonstrated that in the 1348 outbreak, which raged from April to July, burials of female plague victims were equal to those of males (of 146 burials which included 19 children, 69 were male, 69 female and 8 were unknown).[292] Corroboration from the excavation of other Black Death cemeteries is awaited.

The archaeological evidence also provides some surprising and thought-provoking clues about the immediate state and treatment of the dead. The discovery of buckles and other dress accessories indicates that a significant minority of the dead, 3 per cent (24), were clothed when buried (all adults, of which half were men and one-quarter women). The accessories found varied from small platelets of copper to large paired buckles for breeches or trousers (see Fig. 9). Slightly more than half of this group were placed in one of the mass burial trenches, and the obvious conclusion is that the poor souls perished in their houses or in the street, and were gathered up for burial just as they were found.

However, excavations at the Augustinian friary in Hull recovered a range of burials made in the church during the plague, where clear evidence of clothing was abundant, and where the conclusion reached was that these were the well-to-do buried in their best clothes, and in very carefully crafted coffins.[293] Therefore, the temptation to explain the presence of clothing at the London cemetery as a consequence of people being buried in the clothes they died in, should be resisted.

The frequency of coffin use across the whole East Smithfield cemetery contributes further to this issue of preparation and management of the dead. The bodies of more than one-quarter of the dead, 214 (27 per cent), had been placed in wooden coffins before burial, regardless of age or sex. The evidence for this was revealed through the discovery of evenly spaced iron nails around the skeleton, or through the observation of a dark line left by the mainly decayed wood of the coffin sides (so many more coffins may have rotted away entirely). This pattern does not occur anywhere else in excavated medieval Christian cemeteries in Britain,[294] and hints at a specific use of coffins for containing the corrupted dead. This overall figure hides an important distinction between burials made in individual graves, where very nearly one-half were in coffins, and those placed in the mass trenches, where figures averaged at about 11 per cent.[295] This

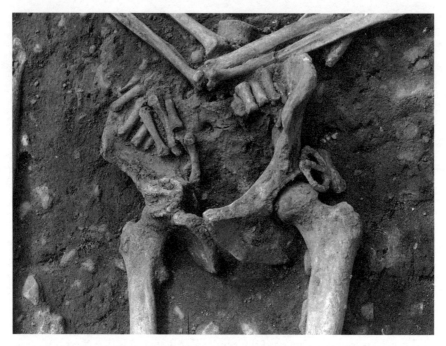

Fig. 9 Detail of the skeleton of a man buried clothed in the East Smithfield cemetery. The partially corroded buckles supporting his leggings can be seen in situ on his hips. (Photograph copyright Museum of London Archaeology)

difference implies a clear distinction between the two groups which will be explored further below.

The use of coffins was absolutely required by some European cities, and while London does not seem to have adopted such a strict approach, some centralised pattern of corporate or civic management of the dead not recorded in documents may be in evidence here. Considering the scale of the mortality and the rates of burial at the other cemeteries, it seems almost certain that a significant temporary industry was required to supply the number of coffins suggested by this figure. Previewing the conclusions on mortality (see Chapter 5), if 27 per cent of all the London dead were buried in coffins, some 285 tons of timber would have been required (based on known medieval coffin sizes, some 9,000 coffins, and a density of oak at around 750kg per m³). It is a great shame that we cannot tell how this massive demand was met, whether through corporate payments to carpenters and joiners, through private purchase, or through the use of crude, home-made structures.

A total of fifteen coffins (7 per cent) were given a dark ashy lining on to which the deceased were laid (see Fig. 10). This group is of national

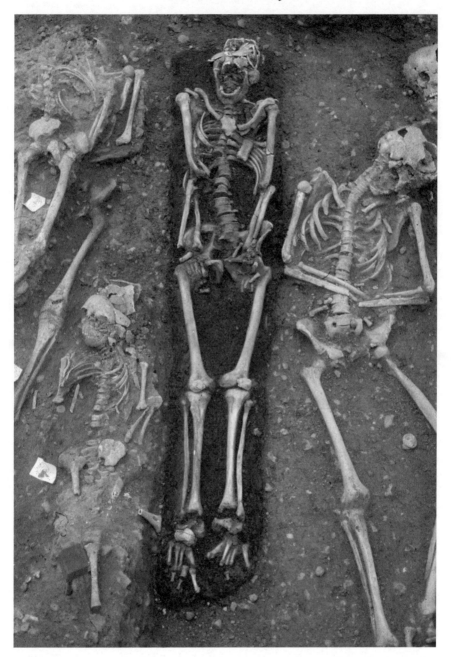

Fig. 10 The burial of a woman in a coffin lined with ash in the East Smithfield cemetery. The coffin has decayed completely but the ash preserves much of its original shape. (Photograph copyright Museum of London Archaeology)

significance, since it represents approximately 30 per cent of all examples of this kind of burial practice in Britain at this time (so far known). The ash, forming a layer perhaps 1cm thick, appears to have been domestic in nature. It contained burned food remains (bone, shell, seeds) and burned pottery fragments. It has been suggested that this was a kind of sponge to absorb putrefaction products and reduce the odour, but the rarity of the rite militates against this; more recently it has been proposed that the material was placed in the coffin at the site of death (usually, therefore, at home) as a symbolic link to the household, and as a means of discouraging the dead from returning home as an undead revenant.[296] If this is right, then even at the height of the disaster, some people at least were taking considerable care over funeral preparations.

Some personal items were recovered from the dead. From around the ankle of one man was recovered a slender strip of chainmail, possibly the remnant of a hem, or perhaps more likely a decorative item. Providing a more dramatic snapshot in the context of this study were the discoveries of two small coin hoards buried with victims (see Fig. 11). Remarkably both skeletons were identifiable, as adult women, probably between the ages of 26 and 35, and buried in coffins.[297] The larger hoard (181 coins) accompanied a woman buried in one of the ash-lined coffins who was probably wearing a belt. The coins were found in two caches broadly divided into silver pennies, which had been stashed in a pouch slung around the neck or under the shoulder, and farthings (with some larger denominations) possibly in a waist pouch. The numismatic evidence of the coins examined indicates a deposit date of between 1344 and 1351.

The smaller hoard, eight silver pennies, had also been kept in some kind of pouch or purse at the waist of the dead woman, and the latest one issued again dated to 1344–51. Together, these coin groups provide our best empirical evidence of the date of the cemetery, but they do a fair bit more than that. The ashy linings of coffins were found in only 2 per cent of all plague burials, so seem not to represent some manner of general disinfectant policy, but rather indicate some other deliberate ritual. In contrast, given the strenuous efforts by the wealthy to ensure through wills that their estate was passed on, and in light of the fact that the burial of money with the dead was extremely rare in medieval England, it seems inconceivable that relatives would deliberately have buried such considerable sums with their owners. The answer probably lies in a combination of haste (represented by the lack of willingness to search and remove the dead woman's clothing and possessions), and deliberate respect and veneration (represented by the securing of a wooden coffin and the careful application of ash lining to its base before the burial).

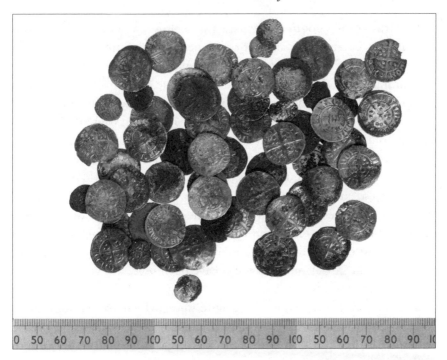

Fig. 11 A selection of the 181 silver coins found with the skeleton of a woman buried in the cemetery at East Smithfield. (Photograph copyright Museum of London Archaeology)

Other evidence does suggest the grimmer side of identifying and collecting burials. One skeleton located in a mass trench was found hunched up in a crouched position, evidence perhaps of rigor mortis and thus of a hurried burial. More telling was the state of the bodies in a small mass burial pit dug towards the eastern edge of the western burial plot. Of eight individuals buried in it, five were adult men, two were teenagers, and one could only be described as adult. At least two of this group were partially disarticulated. This might mean that they had been dug up from elsewhere and transferred here, but far more probably their bodies had lain rotting in deserted buildings or in fields near the city for a considerable time before being found by survivors; their presence in a mass grave hints at some co-ordinated effort to recover bodies.

So we know that in this one cemetery more adults were brought for burial than children, and more men than women; they were, most probably, from the poorer end of the social spectrum; coffins were used for over a quarter of the victims, and some of these show signs both of respect and deliberation, while others suggest haste; and finally, bodies may have come for burial within a single day of death as well as some considerable time afterwards.

How the corpses got to the cemetery is unclear – no London documents describe the day-to-day transport of the dead. Some European cities, such as Florence,[298] saw the emergence of paid collectors and gravediggers. From the chronicles of others (such as William of Dene, see above), it is clear that the disaster was such that people carried their own dead to the graveside. If Robert of Avesbury's figures of up to 200 burials daily in West Smithfield are realistic, one has to consider the involvement of some organising authority capable of ensuring that the flow both of victims and of other city traffic did not become choked. The mass trenches at East Smithfield suggest that there was also an organised collection system not unlike the plague carts of the seventeenth-century outbreaks. The most likely route for the transport of corpses to this was either through Aldgate or by river transport to stairs or jetties east of the Tower; the Postern Gate built some fifty years earlier adjacent to the Tower moat may also have been used, but would not have admitted carts.

The second key aspect of the plague upon which archaeology sheds light is the organisation and use of an emergency cemetery over the plague months. The first thing to note is that two areas were used – the western and eastern plots. Each of the two main burial areas were conspicuously well-ordered. They were split into regular rows (twelve in the west, four in the east) and did not intercut to any significant degree. Within these rows, two principal modes of burial were used: individual graves, and larger, mass burial trenches or pits. We cannot tell from the archaeology whether these areas were used simultaneously or whether when one area was completely filled up, the second was opened, and if so, in which order. We can, however, make some intelligent guesses.

The cemetery was founded in the early months of 1349, probably in February, and was therefore established at a time of high mortality but just before the full height of the plague. It was the last of the three emergency cemeteries to be founded, following the Pardon churchyard and the West Smithfield cemetery, and was thus probably accepting burials which for logistical reasons could be made in neither the local parish or monastic graveyards, nor the two West Smithfield cemeteries. So it is probable that from its first day the cemetery was facing a significant inflow of corpses for burial. The nearest site to the entrance was the western zone, and therefore the earliest burials may have been in the westernmost row of this zone. The first three rows were made up entirely of individual graves, and may thus have been used during February prior to the dramatic spike of mortality implied in March by the wills when will-making doubled and probates tripled. If so, the rate of burial in February might have been about ten per day.

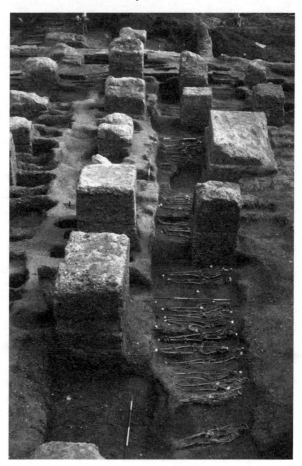

Fig. 12 A view (looking south) of the western mass burial trench at the East Smithfield cemetery during excavation. The square footings are twentieth-century concrete foundations. (Photograph copyright Museum of London Archaeology)

The two mass trenches, one forming the fourth row and the other extending along almost the entire eastern boundary of the cemetery field, are compelling evidence of a step-change in burial rate. The larger, eastern trench probably exceeded 115m in length, while the western one measured about 70m. The latter trench might have contained 600 burials, while that to the east probably held 1,000 or more. Assuming that these trenches were the result of the months of heaviest mortality, March and April, this suggests twenty-five to thirty burials daily, or three per hour in daylight. In the city of Hereford, one parishioner remembered seeing up to twenty bodies buried at the parish church of St Peter in a single day, suggesting such a rate might easily have been reached.[299]

The trenches, about 1.7m deep and 1.9m wide, were both filled very carefully despite the rate at which bodies were supplied. The burials were all set supine in the trench, each body aligned roughly east–west with the head of each corpse laid to the west in accordance with custom (see Fig. 12). Such care shows a particular deliberation even in the face of profound disaster. Each layer of the dead was, exactly as Boccaccio described, covered with a thin capping of soil, and some five layers filled the trenches. There was no archaeological evidence in the two trenches for any 'batching', and it is likely that once the lowest layer was partially complete and sealed in each, further burials were laid down on top, proceeding in sequence until the trenches were full. It seems most likely that ropes were used to lower each corpse into place – the bodies were quite clearly not dumped carelessly out of carts. This same care has been seen in the four mass graves believed to be Black Death graves at the Hospital of the Holy Ghost, Lübeck, Germany, where nearly 700 bodies were found to have been carefully laid, west to east and north to south, in three or four overlapping rows and stacked up to five deep.[300]

Once each mass trench was filled, rows of individual graves followed, six working eastward in the western zone and four working westward along the eastern boundary. These latter four completed the use of the eastern zone. In what precise order the burials took place cannot be ascertained, but there are some clues found in the western zone to suggest that burial may have continued there until the end of the first outbreak and perhaps slightly beyond. Firstly, rows eight and nine saw a reduction in the use of coffins from above 45 per cent to 35 per cent. Then, a third mass trench, 10m long, was dug forming much of the excavated portion of the tenth, western row. Its base stepped up from south to north, suggesting that that was how it was filled, and it held a minimum of fifty corpses.

The distribution of men, women and children was no different from what had gone before, but only two coffins were recorded, both of children under the age of 10 years. Furthermore, the corpse of a teenager had been placed face down, probably accidentally. This trench stopped short of the northern end of the grave row; the last section was occupied by a sizeable grave pit which contained the remains of eight corpses – five men, two teenagers and an unidentified adult. What sets this group aside is the fact that at least three of them were disarticulated before being buried, indicating that they had probably decomposed before burial. It is possible that by this time, the cemetery was being used to bury corpses lost or dumped in the panic of the main outbreak. The last two rows in the western zone were fragmentary, containing five scattered burials each, suggestive of a tail-off of burial activity. An adult in one of these had been buried face down. This is just one interpretation of the evidence and cannot be corroborated; nevertheless, it fits the available facts. It provides a graphic illustration of the manner in which the citizens dealt with the awful physical reality of the disaster, and it brings us, literally, face to face with just a few of the thousands who were slaughtered by the plague in less than six months.

London could not have been alone in identifying such emergency cemeteries, but surprisingly the evidence for other English towns is rather meagre. At Newark, the Archbishop of York authorised the vicar there to buy a piece of land outside the north gate on account of the pressure on burial space. In other towns, parts of existing hospital or monastery cemeteries seem to have sufficed, such as at Worcester, where the cemetery of the hospital of St Oswald, to the north of the city, was pressed into service to supply the deficiency of the cathedral.[301] One curiosity in London is that a huge cemetery already existed outside the walls at St Mary Spital, one of London's largest hospitals. It had functioned as an emergency cemetery a century earlier and again in the great famine of 1315–21, but while a considerable number (1,392) of individual burials of the later thirteenth and fourteenth centuries were excavated,[302] and while mass burial pits were found dating to the twelfth, mid-thirteenth and fifteenth to sixteenth centuries, no such pits were found which could be ascribed to the major fourteenth-century plague outbreaks in London. Unless these have been destroyed by later development, it would appear that the cemeteries at West and East Smithfield were sufficient to manage any superabundance of burials, allowing the hospital to provide single graves for victims that were its responsibility.

The Death Toll

How many thousands died? In London, previous estimates vary, but are worth recounting. Philip Ziegler considered the sum to be about 20–30,000; Naphy and Spicer report estimates between 12,500 and 25,000. Using a novel means of calculation involving known duration and population size, Olea and Christakos considered it reasonable that 50,000 may have died (based on a pre-plague population of 100,000 and assuming a twelve-month duration).[303] We might, in addition, recognise that other historians have entertained the notion of a death toll of 50 per cent or greater in the city,[304] without placing a number to the dead. These estimates have been made without the benefit of the detailed evidence presented earlier and a closer approximation can now be attempted.

There are a number of ways into this question. The first is to look at the ratio of wills made during the plague months in comparison with those made in the years preceding the disease. Rates of will-making demonstrate the citizens' expectation of dying, and, given that large numbers of the wills were probably made at the first sign of infection, it should bear some relevance to the actuality of the mortality. The total of 392 wills drawn up in the nine months from November 1348 to the end of July 1349 (equivalent to a total of 523 wills for a full year), is nineteen times greater than the annual rate of will-making for the twenty years from 1327 prior to the plague. This measure of the expectation of mortality is essentially a measure of the concern of citizens. It might be argued that many more people drew up wills than actually had to, out of fear of a sudden death. This can be checked against the evidence from the other end of the process – the will enrolments of those who definitely did die. Among all those Husting will-makers who encountered the plague and either lived or died, the following categories include:

- Those who made their wills before the outbreak and whose wills were enrolled after its conclusion (n = 16)
- Those who made their wills before the outbreak and whose wills were enrolled during the epidemic months (n = 32)
- Those who made their wills during the epidemic months and whose wills were also enrolled during the epidemic (n = 275)
- Those who made their wills during the epidemic months and whose wills were enrolled after its conclusion (n = 117)

The percentage of people who made their wills during the plague and did not survive it is 70.2 per cent. The percentage of people who made their wills prior to the appearance of the plague but who also did not survive was similar at 68.8 per cent. In other words, there is no apparent surfeit of 'panic' wills: the great majority of those who made wills did so because there was a real need to. Therefore, the rate of increase in the number of wills being made has a direct relationship with the mortality rate.

The number of wills enrolled (572) between 1327 and 1347, perhaps unsurprisingly, is about the same as the number made (587), an average of twenty-seven wills each year. The number enrolled during the nine months of the plague was 307, but we must recall that there is strong evidence for a considerable lag between death and probate dates, and that the court itself was closed during August and September; most of the forty-five wills enrolled in October and November 1349 should, therefore, also be attributed to the main period of the plague. Assuming conservatively that 340 wills were enrolled during the nine-month period, the crude death rate was over sixteen times its annual average. A pre-industrial death rate of about 3.5 per cent per annum for adult males over 20 has been suggested by historical demographers,[305] so we can assume that this percentage of the will-makers would have died anyway during this period, and a figure of 60,000 for the population of London has been argued. Assuming that children of 14 years or less made up 40 per cent of the population (24,000), and that men and women were roughly equal in numbers, then of 18,000 men, 630 would have died per annum. If this percentage was similar for women and children, about 2,100 deaths would have occurred in a normal year. A crude death rate of over sixteen times greater than the norm would indicate a figure of 33,600 dead, or about 56 per cent of the population.

Another way into the problem lies through prosopographical analysis of a group of people whom we know were alive immediately prior to the plague, and whose fates and fortunes can be charted through the documentary evidence beyond the end of the epidemic. Barbara Megson has done just this for a group of 359 wealthy London citizens who were listed for taxation purposes in 1346, and who were alive in 1348 as the plague approached.[306] Her study reveals that some 29 per cent of these richer residents definitely died during the pestilence, and that 38 per cent definitely survived. What is of most interest here is the missing 33 per cent – those who, despite having considerable wealth, simply vanish from the records during the plague and do not, as far as Megson can tell, pick up their businesses and interests once the pestilence had receded. While the simple loss of records is an obvious possibility, the range of documents in which wealthy people might have been named (as witnesses to court cases or transactions, as plaintiffs or defendants in litigation, through wills or receipts of bequests, and so on) is considerable, and so complete disappearance suggests at the least permanent displacement or, more likely, death. If just one-third of the missing group did also die in the epidemic, then the overall implied mortality would be about 40 per cent for the population at large, or about 32,000 dead. If all of the missing perished, then that figure rises to 67 per cent, a level equal to the crude calculation resulting from the rate of will enrolment.

Against another group subject to a similar analysis, a very high death rate may be indicated. Of 118 apprentices enrolled in the Goldsmiths' Company between 1342 and 1346, 106, a frightening 90 per cent, had disappeared from the company records by 1350, many undoubtedly victims of the Black Death.[307] Such a figure requires further examination and research. If substantiated by other apprenticeship records, it would provide a reasonable basis to conclude that the plague was more deadly to the young than to the old.

A further approach is to look at the mortality of the clergy in London. Despite the problems caused by the absence of Bishop Ralph de Stratford's register for the period, there is enough evidence from alternative sources to build a partial picture of this outbreak and indeed subsequent ones (see Chapter 4).[308] Of 111 city churches studied (including St Leonard Shoreditch just beyond the bars), the outcome for sixteen (14.4 per cent) incumbents who were alive at the outbreak are certain. Of this small sample, nine (56.3 per cent) died during the outbreak and seven (43.7 per cent) survived. Some churches lost their incumbents more than once, including St James Garlickehythe and St Mary Woolnoth. A further twenty-one churches display a suspiciously timed change of incumbent in the period 1348–50, which may also have been due to deaths, while at another two the incumbents probably survived. If we were to include these, the death rate for city clergy would rise to 73 per cent. For seventy-two churches we simply do not know who the incumbent was at this particular time. The evidence from this small sample leans towards a mortality rate of above 55 per cent.

Further sources for estimating the death toll is contained in the evidence from the chroniclers and from other contemporary documents. In this regard, Robert of Avesbury's account of the dead being buried in Walter de Mauny's cemetery near West Smithfield is useful. If it is anything more than a proxy for 'a large number', his suggestion of around 200 per day between 2 February and 12 April 1349 implies about 14,000 may have been buried there. In this same period, 192 wills were made. Using the distribution of these wills across the period to establish a ratio, as a means of slanting this average, this figure would produce about 130 burials daily in February, about 210 burials in March, and about 260 burials per day in April. Extrapolating beyond Avesbury's timescale, using this ratio, the number of burials would have dropped to 130 per day in May, 20 in June and below 15 per day in July. These figures would suggest a total of just under 23,000 burials in this cemetery alone. To this needs to be added the victims buried in December and January in the bishop's Pardon churchyard, up to 2,400 buried in the East Smithfield cemetery from February onwards, and all the victims buried in the dozens of parish and monastic cemeteries across the city. A reasonable estimate might be 35,000 dead – about 58 per cent of a population of 60,000. Of course, we have no idea how many non-residents had fled from the surrounding counties towards London (and indeed vice versa), or how many traders and visitors were trapped and engulfed by the disaster.

For the West Smithfield cemetery there is correspondence between de Mauny himself and the Pope suggesting a very large death toll. In early 1352, de Mauny petitioned the Pope, signifying that:

> he, during the epidemic in England, dedicated a place near London for a
> cemetery of poor strangers (*peregrinorum*) and others in which sixty thousand

bodies are buried, and built there a chapel with the licence of the ordinary. He prays for an indulgence of a year and forty days to those who visit the said place on the feasts of Whitsunday, Corpus Christi, and SS Mary Magdalene and Margaret, or who give something to the support of the said chapel and the poor who flock there.

This petition is evidently a replacement for an even earlier one, perhaps of 1351, which appears to have been lost in transit. The papal reply granted on 14 March 1352 gave him licence to endow the chapel and to erect a college of twelve or more chaplains, according to the ordination of the Archbishop of Canterbury and the Bishop of London, and granted the indulgence as requested.[309] However, this letter may also have gone astray on its way back to de Mauny, for the Pope issued a second licence on 12 August 1352, referring in it back to the same huge figure stated by de Mauny, offering 'relaxation … of one year and forty days of enjoined penance to penitents who visit the chapel of the cemetery founded by Walter near London in which are buried more than sixty thousand bodies of those who died of the epidemic – and who give alms for the same'.[310]

The same papal writings were quoted in the early sixteenth century in the Register of the Charterhouse, where the whole basis for the foundation of the cemetery, and after it the monastery, was set out; a figure on a similar scale was quoted by John Stow nearly 250 years after the event, which he read from a stone cross which once stood in the churchyard:

> *Anno Domini 1349. Regnante magna pestilentia consecratum huit hoc coemiterium in quo et infra septa presentis monasterii sepulta fuerunt mortuorum corpora plusquam quinquaginta millia, praeter alia multa abhinc usque presens quorum animabus proprietur deus Amen.*[311]

This translates as: 'The year 1349. A great pestilence reigning, this cemetery was consecrated in which, and within the bounds of the present monastery, were buried more than 50,000 bodies of the dead, as well as many others since then to the present day.' The reference to the monastery (Charterhouse) would date the now-lost cross to at least 1372. A later numerical reference to the dead in this cemetery dates to 1384. A Bull of Urban VI was issued, addressed to the Archbishop of Canterbury, on a petition of Simon, Bishop of London, and Walter de Mauny (who had by this date died). It signalled that the cemetery, in which 'twenty thousand and more dead are buried, in which de Mauny built a chapel, in which certain chaplains were instituted, be transferred to monks of Carthusian order'.[312] While suggesting a more modest figure than de Mauny's own, it still implies a very large cemetery indeed.

What then are we to make of these varying accounts? First, Avesbury has shown himself to be a fairly reliable source on the date of the outbreak in London, and we should therefore not dismiss his claims for burial rates lightly. Second, the issue of de Mauny's claim must be taken still more seriously. De Mauny was a superlative organiser, a seasoned veteran of the French campaigns and, most importantly, someone who had no need of an exaggeration to attract papal support for a new religious foundation. The specification of the cemetery for the use of *peregrinorum* could lie at the heart of this – if the city population was sufficiently bloated by refugees from the surrounding counties, we could entertain such carnage without direct reference to static population estimates for residents alone. Third, we nonetheless acknowledge that while the figures are confused, subject to some change across the later decades of the fourteenth century, they were honoured in an unusual and permanent manner suggesting something quite unique. So fourth, while the figures of 50,000 or 60,000 (equal to up to 100 per cent of our suggested resident population) in one cemetery appears entirely implausible, and while such 'rounded' numbers are often used as a cipher for 'a very large number' in medieval texts, the possibility must be entertained that many thousands, perhaps over 20,000, buried victims still lie somewhere underneath the green spaces of Charterhouse Square and the Charterhouse itself. This is a figure far in excess of previous estimates.[313]

Remarkably, Londoners themselves only ever mention the impact of the plague on the city once in surviving documents. In April 1357, seven years after the event, they petitioned the king for relief from taxation in recognition of the huge sums that the city had lent him to fund his military campaigns in Scotland and France. In the petition they stated that, 'whereas by reason of the death of the richer inhabitants of the City at the time of the pestilence, and their property having fallen into the hand of Holy Church, the City had become impoverished and more than one-third of it empty'.[314] While it is obvious that it would have benefited the civic authorities to enhance any claims of poverty, such a claim as this could quite easily have been checked or challenged – the king's systems for taxation had proved effective at determining who could afford levies such as that of 1346, and the effects of abandonment should have been quite visible – but it was not. If more than one-third of the city was empty in 1357, despite the opportunities provided by seven years of recovery and immigration, the scale of the depopulation could only have been greater. Some evidence of this may exist. Of the ten tenements mentioned as paying for the maintenance of the Great

Conduit in Cheapside, when the two-yearly accounts were delivered in November 1350, three were specifically described as empty, and four of the remainder paid rent during 1348–9 only. Just three were accounted as having returned a rent in the second year (from October 1349 to October 1350).[315]

If more than a third of the city property was indeed empty, the death toll implied is at least equal as a percentage, but probably very much higher, since it would not account for families in other tenements who were reduced but not eradicated by the plague. The smaller villages outside the city were equally badly affected. In the manor and village of Kingsbury, a few miles north-west of the city, there were twelve holdings in the early fourteenth century. In 1350 the manor court learned of the deaths of thirteen people 'at the time of the pestilence'; the holdings were divided among the few survivors, leaving the excess properties empty.[316]

Some later reports managed to exaggerate the impact quite wonderfully. An Icelandic annal of *c.* 1430 claimed that only fourteen persons survived in London after the Great Pestilence of 1349.[317] Written, perhaps, for narrative impact, it is also conceivable that the annal confused general mortality with that among the city's 'ruling' body of the mayor and aldermen of whom there were normally twenty-four. Eight aldermen definitely or probably died during the pestilence, and eighteen were in office at some point during 1349.[318] The overlap caused by new aldermen replacing plague victims is not clear, but the numbers would be about right. The indication is around 40 per cent mortality.

Drawing on the grounds of the wills, documentary evidence and prosopographical evidence, this analysis makes a solid case that over 50 per cent, and possibly more than 60 per cent, of the will-makers and tax-payers of the citizenry perished. Such figures seem extraordinary, but similarly catastrophic levels are suggested both within other English urban centres, in rural localities, and in Continental towns and cities. In Oxford, an average of 1.6 wills per annum was enrolled between 1320 and 1348, a figure which jumped to fifty-seven (thus thirty-six times greater) in 1349; in Colchester, 110 wills were enrolled during 1348–9, almost twenty-five times the annual average for the previous twenty years; and in Lincoln, 105 wills enrolled in 1349 represented a figure of thirty times the average for fifty-three other years between 1315 and 1376. In York and Norwich in 1349, over three times more entries to the freedom of each city were recorded than the average number for previous decades which, while not providing a ratio, certainly indicates the opportunities and needs presented by severe mortality.[319] At Canterbury, about two-thirds of the taxable population included in returns for 1346–9 disappeared from the records by 1351–2.[320]

In rural localities previous syntheses have identified mortality rates of over 50 per cent on twenty-eight Durham priory manors with a range of 30–78 per cent;[321] 40–46 per cent on Halesowen manor, Worcestershire; 50–60 per cent in Coltishall, Norfolk; 49 per cent on Cottenham manor, Cambridgeshire; 45 per cent in mid-Essex communities; and 45–55 per cent in Walsham-le-Willows, Suffolk.[322] Manorial tenants of the Bishop of Worcester in the West Midlands suffered losses ranging from 19 to 80 per cent. Analyses of eleven of the Bishop of Winchester's manors in Hampshire show a loss of tenants ranging from 59 to 100 per cent, with an average of 76 per cent. An innovative study of landless men working seventeen manors of the Abbot of Glastonbury in the West Country found an average mortality rate of 57 per cent.[323] Contemporary manorial assessments made as part of inquisitions post mortem of major landholders include eight survivors of fourteen cottars (43 per cent mortality) at Kidlington (Oxon); four of eight bond tenants (50 per cent) at Titchmarsh (Northants); six of thirteen villeins (54 per cent) at Stanton Harcourt (Oxon); six of twenty-four bondsmen (75 per cent) at Ashby David (Northants); and 100 per cent losses at East Morden (Dorset), Basildon (Berks), Ampthill (Beds) and Todworth (Wilts).[324]

Further afield, some Continental examples offer similar evidence. In France, the town of Givry has a superb set of burial registers which run through the plague (July to October 1348). Annual burial rates pre-plague were twenty-three per annum on average. At 3.5 per cent male deaths per annum, this would have yielded a population of around 650–700 adults, so a population of perhaps 1,100 including children. In the four months of the plague, a total of 626 burials were made in the town's cemetery, or about 57 per cent of the population. The lay confraternity of San Francesco in Orvieto, Italy, also has an excellent burial register backed up by a matriculation list of entries. From this it has been calculated that nearly two-thirds of the community, dwelling in all parts of the city, perished. In Siena, Italy, perhaps just a little smaller than London's population (*c.* 50,000 in the city itself), the death rate was probably as much as 50 per cent; while the much smaller town of San Gimignano probably saw 58.7 per cent. Perpignan suffered between 58 and 68 per cent mortality based on the analysis of the deaths of notaries in that town.[325]

While the value of these assessments is limited by the nature of the evidence, the range of approaches, the variety of the sources and the general consistency of the outcomes all appear to indicate that a mortality rate of 55 or even 60 per cent or more in London seems quite defensible. However, such a death rate begs basic questions: how could the city regain its feet so quickly and carry on functioning if nearly two in three residents were dead? What, therefore, needs consideration is the immediate impact that the 1348–9 disaster had on the city and survivors.

Some Immediate Impacts: 1350–60

The 1348–9 pestilence was the greatest of a succession of outbreaks of disease that rocked the city during Edward III's reign and contributed to an extended and very significant reduction in the population. Studies elsewhere have tended to consider the broader impact of events across this period, especially on the national economy and London's place within it, but there were other impacts that might be viewed as a specific legacy of this first catastrophe. Medieval Londoners (indeed people across Europe) had never suffered a cataclysm even remotely on this scale before, and certainly not one whose origin was placed by their own church leaders in the hands of their God and in response to their sins. Under the circumstances, we should be able to detect some kind of communal reaction, in public and private life, in social spheres and in people's attitudes, to religion and death. An in-depth review of all the available evidence for the decade lies beyond the reach of this volume, but we can identify some key impacts.

The impact with the greatest publicity was the effect of the huge death toll on the nation's economic fortunes. At the first Parliament held since the outbreak of the plague, in February 1351, the king himself acknowledged the visible signs of this impact:

> he is informed that the peace of the land is not well kept, and that there are very many other crimes and faults which need to be redressed and amended, as shown by maintenance of parties and complaints in the localities, and also … servants and labourers who are not willing to work and labour as they are accustomed.[326]

The commons were more forthright still. In their petition, they noted:

> how his commonalty is greatly ruined and destroyed by this pestilence, because of which cities, boroughs and other vills and hamlets throughout the land have decayed … and many which used to pay the tax of the tenth and fifteenth and other charges granted to him in aid of his war are completely depopulated. And now, because of their deaths, this new conditional tax, which is assessed at the same sum on those who have survived, destroys and ruins them to such an extent that they can scarcely stay alive.[327]

There were other, more subtle issues triggered by the plague, national in scope, but certainly of interest to the city's survivors. One such was the matter of the legal status of children born overseas, and it is surely no coincidence that this was again on the parliamentary agenda. It no doubt reflects the high level of mobility and migration that ensued as survivors of the epidemic began to assert their rights to estates, or to take advantage of new opportunities. Edward himself was sensitive to the potential impact, and sought to close loopholes:

> some people were in doubt whether the children born in overseas parts outside the allegiance of England should be able to demand inheritance within the same allegiance or not, on account of which a petition was formerly put in the parliament held at Westminster in the seventeenth year of our lord the king [1343–4] and was not at such time completely agreed, our said lord the king, wishing that all doubts and uncertainties were removed and the law in this case declared and clarified.[328]

That London experienced a considerable influx of people immediately following the plague is in little doubt – we have already seen the king's empowerment in late December 1349 of the city sheriffs to keep the peace amid the 'great concourse of aliens and denizens to the city and suburbs, now that the pestilence is stayed'. Despite this inward migration, however, many of its buildings – as many as one-third – remained empty for several years, as claimed in the parliamentary petition for tax relief in 1357. The opportunity for survivors and migrants to improve, or obtain for the first time, landholding and especially trading sites by entering such empty properties may have proved too great a temptation for some. Examination of the Possessory Assizes, the court that dealt with disputes over property ownership, between the years 1340 and 1348, shows an average of about eight cases per year. Fifteen cases were held in the three months alone following the resumption of the court in November 1349 and (following a further break between February 1350 and October 1351) a further thirty-three were held in the nine months to July 1352. Clearly the legal complexities of establishing true title led to considerable argument and arbitration.

The shortage of labour in the city had already led to the Ordinance of Labourers being issued in 1349; this was repeated in 1350 as a result of 'the damages and grievances which the good folks of the City, rich and poor, have suffered and received within the past year, by reason of masons, carpenters, tilers and all manner of labourers, who take immeasurably more than

they have been wont to take'.[329] In 1351 the wages pressure remained sufficiently high for the commons to take their grievance to the king:

> since the pestilence labourers are unwilling to work, to the great misfortune
> of the people, and to take for their labour what was agreed by our lord the
> king and his council, and they have no regard for fines or redemptions, but go
> day to day from bad to worse. May it please our lord the king that corporal
> punishment with redemptions shall be imposed on them when they shall be
> attainted in due manner.[330]

The ordinance was enshrined in law, becoming the Statute of Labourers.
However, London was, for the king at least, far from efficient in enforcing the statute. Following further complaints to Parliament about prices in
London in 1354, suggestions for administrative remedies omitted mention of
those supposedly appointed to enforce the statute, the justices of labourers.
A year later, enquiry by the Exchequer revealed that no one in London knew
whether or not there were any such justices. Pressure forced the mayor to act
and by 1357 the Letter Book provides significant details of those being prosecuted under the statute. Between 1 August 1357 and 29 September 1359, the
City Letter Books record that seventy-four men, almost all apparently in the
construction industry (carpenters, tilers, masons etc.), were fined an average
of nearly 1s 6d each for a total of £5 7s 4d.[331]

There are numerous examples of the extreme pressure exerted on the
artificial wages ceiling. Among the swiftest and more extreme changes in
wages were the costs of the harvest. The manorial accounts survive for
the Westminster Abbey manors of Knightsbridge, Hyde (now covered by
Hyde Park) and Ebury (modern Mayfair, Belgravia and Pimlico), and from
these, the costs of managing the harvest have been calculated.[332] Reaping
and binding 1 acre was charged at 8.39 pence on average across the three
London manors before the plague; immediately afterwards, this figure had
rocketed to 14.28 pence, an increase of 70 per cent. Threshing and win-
nowing one-quarter each of wheat, barley and oats before the plague cost
7.41 pence; immediately afterwards this had risen to 13.02 pence, a 75 per
cent rise. Day-wages on the three manors also increased in the ten years up
to 1359. Notwithstanding the Statute of Labourers, skilled craftsmen such as
carpenters, thatchers and tilers saw their wages rise between 26 and 38 per
cent, while general labourers enjoyed a 97 per cent rise.[333]

The four servants of the church receiving board-wages at Westminster
Abbey (wages in lieu of food and board) collected 8d per week before the
plague and for four years afterwards, but their wage rose to 1s in 1354, up

50 per cent, while the annual stipend paid to the chandler for transporting candle wax and sconces from London to the abbey rose from 6s 8d to 10s.[334] It has been suggested that London may have been exceptional in its response to the statute in comparison to the rest of the kingdom, possibly as a result of a generally higher cost of living, and that the civic authorities effectively ignored both ordinance and statute.[335]

Prices of basic commodities rose sharply as a result of disruption to the established markets. Wool prices were the least affected, rising by about 10 per cent over the decade, but prices for one-quarter of wheat rose as high as 16s in 1352 with an average of over 7s across the decade, as compared with 4s 4d in the previous decade.[336] The price of salt more than doubled from 3s 3d to 6s 7d a quarter, and iron was claimed in 1354 to be four times its pre-plague price, prompting loud calls to the king in Parliament for a cap on exports and pricing:

> his commons pray: that whereas he has a great scarcity of iron in the land because he has not put any definite price on the same, and a great part of the same is exported out of England; and whereas a stone of iron used to be sold for 3d before the pestilence, it is now sold for 12d, to the great damage and impoverishment of the said commonalty; may it please his lordship to ordain that no iron shall be exported out of the realm on penalty of forfeiture of the same, and that a definite price shall be put on iron, in alleviation of the afore-said misfortunes.[337]

Labourers were not the only kind of manpower that was thin on the ground. In the guilds, eight wardens of the Cutlers' Company, six of the Hatters and four of the Goldsmiths were swept away, indicative of the impact on the skilled trades in the city. The pepperers lost an estimated 34 per cent of their fraternity.[338] The effect was therefore likely to have been very apparent as migrants or semi-skilled apprentices filled the gaps, and it may have been this which prompted several guilds to issue (or re-issue) their articles and ordinances in 1350.[339] One case readily demonstrates the squeezes of simultaneous skill loss and price rises during this period. On 28 June 1350 a bill of complaint issued by the Saddlers' Company was read in which the company of Fusters of the City (makers of wooden saddle-frames) were charged with price-fixing and agreeing not to sell a saddle-tree:

> [formerly] costing 6d or 7d, for less than 2s or 30d, although the wood of which it was made cost only 3d. They complained further that the Fusters had agreed not to take any apprentices, with the intention of restricting the number of

their mistery, so that they could control prices. They also agreed to sell their saddle-bows to foreigners, if they could not obtain their price among citizens, and they were about to buy a charter from the King restricting the trade to those persons who were now confederated, which would result in the decrease of the mistery. A similar confederacy had formerly existed among the lorimers in copper, of whom there were now only two left to serve the whole people.

The claim was denied and in early July it came to court. William Pykerel, on behalf of the saddlers, proposed that due to the impact of the pestilence during the last two years, a new scale of charges for goods supplied by the fusters to the saddlers should be adopted, 'that all saddle-trees should be of good material, that the Fusters should take apprentices, and that they should not sell to foreigners so long as there was a sale among citizens'. The fusters prepared a counter-proposal, in which they said:

> that they could not find apprentices or serving men to help them, and that at a time when they needed more comfort in the matter of food and clothing, conditions were so evil that the gallon of beer cost 2*d* instead of 1*d*, and other necessaries had also risen in like proportion. Consequently they could not sell at the prices suggested by the Saddlers, since they would be spending more in a year than they could earn in three ... They prayed the Mayor and Aldermen to accept a schedule of prices for certain kinds of saddle-trees.

The upshot was an (increased) arbitrated price structure agreed by both sides.[340] It is significant that the case refers to just two lorimers (copper-smiths) remaining.

Clergy, too, were charging high stipends to serve, and many were exchanging their current livings for better paid ones. Senior clergy were outraged at this development, and on 28 May 1350 the Archbishop of Canterbury issued the decree Effrenata seeking to cap the level of stipends. It was sent first to Ralph Stratford, Bishop of London, as dean of the province with a request to enforce it in his own diocese, to make a list of runaway priests and to inform the other bishops of its provisions – he was to report back before 8 September. This measure clearly had less effect than was intended, for on 18 February 1352, the archbishop had again to write to Stratford complaining that priests cared more for money than for the safety of their souls, and that in the diocese of London there were a large number of runaway clergy who were under ecclesiastical sentences for disobedience to the Effrenata.[341]

The problem was not one to be solved easily, although several surviving bishops' registers attest to increased recruitment and promotion (sadly we have no London evidence for this activity until 1362, since the bishops' registers for the relevant years are missing). Henry Knighton's chronicle makes a scathing attack on the quality of the replacements, noting that 'within a short time a very great multitude whose wives had died of the plague rushed into holy orders. Of these many were illiterate and, it seemed, simply laymen who knew nothing except how to read to some extent.' Many of those ordained jockeyed both during and after the plague for better livings. William Langland spelled out his oft-quoted commentary on the rush to 'sing for simony' in London at the expense of impoverished rural parishes.[342] However exaggerated this may have been for poetic impact, examples such as a vicar indicted under the Statute of Labourers for attempting to charge the extortionate price of 5s or 6s to perform a marriage indicate that profiteering was taking place.[343]

The pestilence had a profound effect on religious orders as well as secular clergy, and while specific numbers for London's religious houses are unclear in this post-plague decade, it is apparent that many monks and canons fled their convents. Apostasy peaked dramatically in the middle decades of the fourteenth century, probably as a result of 'unimaginable stresses and strains experienced in many religious communities, especially perhaps the small ones, as a consequence of catastrophic mortality'.[344]

Westminster Abbey is better documented than any other religious house in the London area, and we can gain a glimpse of the impact of the plague on its fortunes. By September 1353 the community stood at just twenty-nine monks and the abbot, compared with a pre-plague total of fifty or more monks.[345] The infirmarer's office was significantly affected by the plague, his income being halved immediately. His responsibilities included the management of day-patients (those who continued to sleep in the dormitory but were excused from their normal daily duties for a period of a few days to come to the infirmary for rest and treatment) and in-patients (those who entered the infirmary long term on account of their debilitation). Partial and intermittent accounts surviving from before the plague can be compared with those in the years immediately after, and it has been suggested that the plague brought about a significant shift in the frequency of each type of patient.

In the half-century before the plague, 602 instances of day care were recorded along with 263 in-patients; in the three years from September 1350 to August 1353, sixteen day-patients were treated, compared with twenty-one in-patients. The former also now visited the infirmary as day-patients for consecutive periods lasting nearly twice as long as before (a median of 7.5 days per event as opposed to 4 previously). This has been interpreted as a squeeze on day-patient care, with the bar for admission being set higher than previously, either by the impact of the plague itself in leaving behind only the fitter monks who had less need of access to day-patient care, or perhaps more likely as a result of the severe shortage of manpower available to treat the day-patients, along with the reduction in available funding to do so.[346] If such a shift in practice embedded itself following this and later plague outbreaks, it may have had a direct influence on evolving arrangements of monastic infirmaries, a subject to which we will return in the concluding chapter.

The sacrist's office at Westminster was probably least affected by the plague. By 1354–5 the income had recovered to over £224, of which £30 came from St Edward's shrine and £15 from the old altar of St Mary by the north door. This speaks of a very significant popular desire to make offerings within the church, and some special indulgence had probably been obtained in connection with the abbey's relics, since criers of London were employed to advertise the terms (although what these were is not known). The specific sum offered to St Mary's altar seems especially significant in this regard: the Virgin's role in the salvation of the Christian congregation was believed to be vitally important during the plague. The loss of religious persons from the convent did have clear impacts on the liturgical cycle despite this income: from the accounts of the wardens of the Lady Chapel and altars, it is clear that in 1351 only three of the five principal feasts of the Blessed Virgin Mary were marked by a High Mass, and it was not until a decade later that the full five were reinstated.[347]

The impact of the plague may also be seen in the approach of the abbey in discharging its charitable obligations to the poor. When on 28 November 1290 Eleanor of Castile was buried at Westminster Abbey, a foundation was set up to provide penny doles to the poor coming on each anniversary of her death to the gates. Until the 1340s, the total sum often exceeded £100 annually, providing for a minimum of 12,000–15,000 (and conceivably above 24,000) poor people gathering at the abbey gates in late November. However, for a century after the plague, the largest sum was to be £25 3s 4d. This change is underlined by an analysis of the sums distributed through the abbey's almonry, lying to the west of the abbey church alongside Tothill Street. Here, a minimum average of £177 per annum was distributed to the poor up to 1349, while the figure for the second half of the fourteenth century was down 43.5 per cent to around £100. There were clearly fewer of the poor around, but we may also detect the impact of the Ordinance and Statute of Labourers. In addition, there was a change in ideology which focused far more on the 'deserving' poor, and a linked shift in charitable emphasis away from the casual poor towards residential recipients, not just at Westminster but in an increasing number of hospitals across the country.[348]

Measuring the impact on other religious houses is difficult as, by and large, good documentary evidence does not survive. The house of the Crutched Friars had thirteen inmates in December 1350, compared with a maximum of twenty in the first half of the fourteenth century. The Franciscan friary near Newgate held ninety friars in 1336, and while there is no direct evidence for the immediate post-plague figures, by the last decade of the fourteenth century, resident numbers may have been as low as forty-three.[349] Hospitals, perhaps inevitably, fared the worst and we have already noted the almost complete depopulation of St James Westminster and St Thomas Southwark. The leper hospital of St Giles lost its warden, Thomas de Kirkeby, and three of the sisters, Cecilia de Shobyndon, Edith de Ispania and Christina Sencler,[350] and the plague may have been the catalyst for a detailed examination of the hospital just a few years later. In March 1354 the mayor and commonalty petitioned the king and council regarding its purpose and management. Reminding the king that the hospital had been founded, generously endowed and effectively managed by elected London citizens from the twelfth century, they noted that Edward I had handed the hospital over to the order of leper knights of St Lazarus, based in Burton Lazars, and complained that since then, the lepers had been ousted from the hospital to be replaced by brothers and sisters of the order, 'who were not diseased, contrary to the will of the donors aforesaid and to the great danger of healthy persons intermingling with the said lepers'. The petition requested that 'poor diseased folk of the city be restored to the said hospital'.

The house, comprising one warden, three brothers, two sisters, two secular priests and fourteen poor lepers at the end of 1354, is said to have suffered 'by fire and by pestilence'.[351] Other matters of health and sanitation were raised in 1354, this time by the king over the area of the Fleet prison and its neighbourhood. Edward complained to the city authorities about the potential harm of the stench from butchery and the cleaning of entrails on a wharf near to the prison, drawing strength from an earlier petition by the prior of St John Clerkenwell, who also considered the threat to be potentially injurious to the health of the prisoners (and who coincidentally had land interests nearby). A year later, the king commissioned an inquiry into the construction of unlicensed privies over the Fleet Ditch surrounding the prison, and the filth accumulating from these and several tanneries discharging into it. The city authorities conceded the issue and in 1355 provided another place for the butchers near the wall of the Dominican friary on the bank of the Thames.[352]

The problem persisted, however, and in 1357 the king issued a further order to the city, stating that in past times the city's streets and lanes had been accustomed to regular cleaning but that now, filth accumulated there and on the banks of the Thames, 'which, if tolerated, great peril, as well to the persons dwelling within the said city, as to the nobles and others passing along the said river, will, it is feared, ensue'. The mayor was therefore to ensure that the city was kept clean on 'pain of heavy forfeiture'.[353] The link between these concerns and the pestilence itself is not explicit, but the 'great peril' would have raised but one spectre in the minds of those hearing the king's words. We have already seen Edward's concern over the filth in the city streets at the height of the first plague, and we will see once more worries about the stench of rotting refuse during the second and third outbreaks. It does seem likely that a new sensitivity to the urban environment was engendered through fear of the disease recurring.

If there was a suspicion that the threat to life had not fully receded, it was probably correct. It looks as if there was a significant dip in fertility, with families becoming smaller, and at the same time an increase in the likelihood of childhood mortality, neither of which was conducive to a rapid replenishment of the population. There is, of course, no census data, but a partial idea of family sizes in the fourteenth century in general has been advanced, based on the information contained in wardship cases brought before the city courts.[354] From 1309 to 1348, the average number of children per family suggested by this calculation was 1.79. In the first decade after the Black Death, this figure dropped to just 1.5 and remained significantly lower throughout the fourteenth century. This pattern is generally supported (but with rather lower figures) through an examination of the number of direct offspring mentioned in the Husting wills. Between 1 January and 31 October 1348, a total of thirty-four will-makers identified forty-nine children as beneficiaries, an average of 1.44 per testator. The male-to-female ratio was 1.08 for these children.

During the key plague months, from 1 November 1348 until 31 July 1349, a further 392 wills were drawn up which identified a total of 428 child beneficiaries, an average of 0.92 children per will-maker. The male-to-female ratio had increased to 1.12. For the decade from August 1349 to July 1359, 132 will-makers made bequests to 125 children, an increase to 1.05 per will-maker. The male-to-female ratio increased to 1.27. These figures show just a partial picture, but it does seem likely that the trend was downward. In terms of increasing mortality, analysis of the wardships shows that between 1309 and 1348, 18 per cent of orphans of both sexes who were entered into wardship (between 7 and 10 years old) did not survive to come of age (at 21). This rose very significantly to 27 per cent between 1349 and 1398.[355]

Examination of the male heirs of wealthier merchant families shows a similar pattern but suggests a slightly greater risk for this group. Between 1318 and 1347, 23 per cent of merchant sons orphaned as youngsters died before coming of age. Between 1348 and 1377, this figure rose sharply to 33 per cent.[356] While the sex ratio of the children mentioned in the Husting wills is not a reliable indicator of the wider demographic structure of the city, it is of interest because it hints at one of two things: either there were more male children surviving the plague (or being born) than female, or there was an increase in the desire to name boys as beneficiaries at the expense of girls.

The pattern of will-making changed in other immediate ways. At a basic level, the number of people both making and enrolling wills at the Husting court fell from a pre-plague level of around twenty-eight wills per annum to half that figure – an annual average of 12.4 wills were drawn up and 15.6 enrolled between 1351 and 1360. While obviously indicative of the mortality level, it may also reflect the concentration of property into fewer hands. The nature of the wills also changed. People began to specify their burial locations in much greater detail, selecting not only the church or monastery, but often specifying the churchyard, chancel, porch or chapel that they desired as their resting place. Although known from as early as 1275, the specification of burial location was very rare in the wills until the 1330s, and the first plague seemed not to have made much of a difference to this initially. For the period January 1347 to the end of October 1348, thirty of sixty-six (about 45 per cent) Husting wills drawn up expressed a preference. Of 392 wills which were made in the key plague months, between 1 November 1348 and 1 August 1349, 182 (a comparable 46 per cent) did so. The first plague, therefore, did not seem to have instantly modified Londoners' approach to their own resting places. Once survivors had had a chance to take stock, however, the frequency increased dramatically. In the period from 1 September 1349 to 31 December 1359, nearly 74 per cent of citizens specified their choice of burial location (99 out of 134 wills made). Examples include John atte Bataylle, a weaver, who specified burial in the processional way within the church of St Giles Cripplegate in 1352; and John Edward, a butcher, who chose the chapel of St Mary within the church of St Leonard Eastcheap.[357] It seems entirely probable that this upsurge occurred in response to the chilling memories of vast plague pits, lost relatives and uncounted, unmarked graves.

London's pool of intellectual and artistic skill must have been dealt a severe blow. The city's administrators and elected officials had suffered with at least thirteen aldermen known to have died in the first outbreak[358] leaving both a requirement and an opportunity for new blood to prove itself in the complex political and economic world of the city. Adam Fraunceys rose from alderman to mayor within one year (1352) without holding office as sheriff first, and this speed of promotion was partly due to the effect of the pestilence.[359] Architects and designers were killed, such as William Ramsey, who designed St Paul's chapter house and cloisters; his successor, John atte Greene; and Walter le Bole, master mason at Westminster.[360] Metalsmiths clearly suffered and a quick scan of the occupations noted in the Husting wills shows that fifteen goldsmiths, two bell-founders and two pewterers perished, alongside numerous craftsmen working and trading leather, wood and cloth. It has been suggested that the king's decision to impress glaziers to complete the windows at St Stephen's chapel Westminster may have been because of the dearth of skilled craftsmen.[361]

Almost certainly, more than half of London's resident population had been killed or displaced, buildings stood empty, trade was affected, and social and economic networks had been transformed. The psychological scars of such a profoundly shocking experience are not easy to establish, but we can detect immediate shifts in approaches to bequests through wills, suggesting that the way people saw the world had fundamentally altered. These changes were to be more deeply embedded in the city (and indeed the country) as it was rocked by no fewer than three further outbreaks before 1377, each one amplifying the impact of the last. The most significant of these later visitations was the *pestis secunda* of 1361, but chroniclers also pointed out widespread outbreaks in 1368–9 and 1375, and it is to these subsequent and less well known pestilences that we now turn.

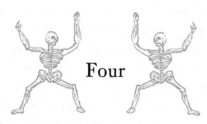

Four

PESTILENCE IN LATER FOURTEENTH-CENTURY LONDON

Pestis Secunda, *1361*

Secunda mortalitas. Eodem anno mortalitas generalis oppressit populum que diceba-tur Pestis Secunda. Et moriebantur tam maiores quam minores, et maxime iuvenes et infantes.

The second mortality. That same year a widespread mortality, known as the Second Plague, overwhelmed the people. And the great were killed along with the masses, and especially infants and the young.[362]

Anno xxxv (Edward III): And that same yere men, bestys, treys, and howsys were smyght fervently with lytthenyge, and sodenly i-peryschyde. And they fonde in mennys lyckenys splatt men goyng in the waye.

The 35th year (Edward III): And in that same year, men, beasts, trees and houses were smitten violently with lightning and suddenly perished. And fiends in the likeness of men accosted men as they went their way.[363]

Mesme celle ane fuist la secunde pestilence parmy Engleterre la quel fuist appelle la mortalites des enfauntz.

That same year was the second pestilence in the country of England which was called the mortality of the infants.[364]

Such are the chronicles of the events in 1361, but there is a short foreword to this second disaster in which London may have been visited by some kind of outbreak as early as the autumn of 1360. The Chronicle of the Greyfriars of King's Lynn notes: 'In that year [1360] began a plague among Londoners at about the feast of St Michael, where at first infants died in huge numbers.'[365] This lone reference has, perhaps, the feel of a scribal error about it, and might best be conflated with the main outbreak of 1361, but we cannot actually tell. Apart from the fact that a disease initially affecting the young would be unlikely to be well represented in evidence from wills, the wills themselves do not survive for this specific time: roll 88 of the Husting court, dating to between January 1360 and February 1361, is missing.[366] Of the wills drawn up in 1360, we have just ten which happened to be proved in March 1361 or later when the sequence resumes, and none of these offer any clue about such an outbreak. Additionally, among charters from Colchester, Essex, is one from 1410 which notes a will from 34 Edward III (so January 1360 to January 1361) at the time of the *secunda pestilencia*.[367] It remains possible, therefore, that a plague, one which affected the young, did strike the city in the last months of 1360.

There is, however, no doubt about the events of the following spring. The greyfriars of Lynn may be quoted again:

> and after the next Easter following [April 1361], men and women died in great multitudes ... In that year the plague raged in the southern parts of England with great mortality among children, youths and the wealthy. This plague was however much less serious than that which had befallen thirteen years before.[368]

This report is backed up by most other contemporary chroniclers. As well as Henry Knighton (above), the Anonimalle Chronicle called it the mortality of children, and states that several people of high birth and a great number of children died.

A striking aspect of the reports was that not only was this outbreak apparently killing the young, but it was disproportionately killing men. Higden's Polychronicon, claiming that it actually started in London, called it a 'great pestilence of men ... killing many men but few women'; Walsingham also asserted that the disease devoured men rather than women. John of Reading's chronicle stated that 'this year the mortality was particularly of males, who were devoured in great numbers by the pestilence'; and the chronicle of Louth Abbey described 'a mortality of men, especially of boys'.[369]

The anonymous Canterbury Chronicle provides us with some description of the outward symptoms of the disease:

> Children and adolescents were generally the first to die, and then the elderly. Members of religious orders and parish clergy and others died suddenly

without respect of persons when the first spots and the other signs of death appeared on their bodies, as on the bodies of the victims everywhere. Many churches were then left unserved and empty through lack of priests. The plague lasted for more than four months in England.[370]

In contrast to the first epidemic, the course of the 1361 plague across England and indeed Europe has yet to be clearly established – certainly there seem to be few warning references in clerical correspondence, so it may well be that the outbreak originated in England and possibly in London as the Lynn greyfriars and the Canterbury Chronicles maintain. The Husting wills for 1361 do show the Canterbury Chronicle to be absolutely correct regarding the date, and the outbreak in the city can probably be dated to as precise a time as the second half of April (see Fig. 13).[371] A total of fifteen wills were drawn up in that month, nine of them in its last twelve days. To put this into perspective, in the decade from January 1350 to December 1359, a total of 129 wills were drawn up (which were eventually enrolled in the Husting court), meaning the yearly average had been exceeded in one month.

Agnes, the unmarried daughter of cordwainer Richard Sorel, living in the parish of St Michael-le-Quern, is probably the earliest identifiable victim: her will dated 22 April and was proved in Husting just four days later. Another early victim may have been Margaret Cadoun, an orphan and minor whose death on 25 April was reported by her guardian, Richard Russell, when he came to recover money left in trust for her.[372] Enrolments during the first two weeks of the plague totalled eight, seven of which had been drawn up before the outbreak. Of these, one was for Alan de Scarnyngge, a clerk at Holy Trinity priory, Aldgate, who had lived through the first plague and who left 10s for his daughter's wedding, to be arranged by the prior for whom he had worked.[373] Perhaps significantly, the king also issued orders strongly reminiscent of those made during the first outbreak, closing the ports on 30 April to any except merchants.[374]

In May, the number of wills drawn up leapt to twenty-nine. Among these was the will of Roger de Codyngton, dated to 29 May, who specified burial in the church of 'St Mary of the New Work' in Aldersgate, the chapel founded by de Mauny in the West Smithfield plague cemetery.[375] The chapel and cemetery were the subject of intensive planning at this dangerous time, evidence of which comes from an agreement drawn up on 9 May 1361 between de Mauny himself and Michael de Northburgh, Ralph Stratford's successor as Bishop of London. The agreement, relating to the foundation of both chapel and cemetery, was of such importance that it was recited verbatim in the early sixteenth-century Register of the Charterhouse. It said:

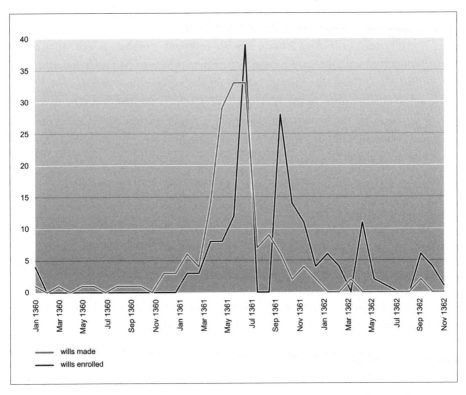

Fig. 13 Wills made and enrolled in the Husting court between January 1360 and November 1362, providing clear evidence of the peak between April and October 1361. (Source: CHW, Vol. 2)

Walter de Mauny received the said bishop as his first associate for the foundation and advowson and building of the church of the Annunciation of Our Lady without London beside Smethefeld ... It was also agreed that the beginning of this foundation was, during the pestilence which was [in 1349] and is in the present, to bury here in the cemetery the bodies of all Christians, especially of the City of London, who wish to be buried there, of rich as well as of poor ... and as well without regard to the pestilence as during the pestilence, but especially during the pestilence.[376]

It is important in the context of this study because it specifically refers to further burials in the Smithfield cemetery during this second outbreak: the emergency cemetery was being pressed into service once more. De Northburgh's will, dated 23 May, in reinforcing the agreement, further indicated his intention to found a Carthusian monastery on the site of the Newchurchehawe, for which he bequeathed the very considerable sum of £2,000. De Mauny issued a letter patent just a day after de Northburgh's will was drawn up, notifying that:

an agreement having been arranged between him and Sir Michael de Northburgh, bishop of London, with reference to the church of the Annunciation of Our Lady without Smethefeld, which he had lately founded, it had pleased him that the said bishop for the advancement of that church, and of the religious house [Charterhouse], which they both intended to found, and for the benefit of the said place, might henceforth act as he, the said bishop, thought fit without hindrance from him, or without obtaining his consent, if absent.[377]

Such plans were, however, going to suffer a setback: de Northburgh was to die in just four months' time.

Work on royal projects was not to be set aside despite the worsening situation, and as de Scarnyngge's will was being copied into the Husting rolls, the king was appointing Richard de Normanton, clerk of the king's works in the Tower of London, with funds to source sufficient workmen, to accommodate himself in the Tower and to convey materials there. Thomas Chamberleyn likewise was charged with the delivery of stone, timber, lime, tiles and other necessaries for the king's works in Westminster Palace and the Tower of London, and carriage for the same, to be paid for by the hands of the king's surveyor, William de Lambheth.[378] Edward appears to have shown urgency in the matter of completing one particular royal religious project among the several he was progressing at this time, and perhaps for good reason. St Mary Graces, founded on the site of the Holy Trinity plague cemetery near the Tower, remained substantially incomplete.

On 17 March 1361 Edward appointed John Cory, the clerk who had consolidated the land for the cemetery in 1349, and John de Tiryngton, a master mason, 'to take twenty-four carpenters, masons, tilers and other workmen' for works at the abbey. The king also provided royal protection for the workmen, wishing 'to hasten on the works as much as possible'.[379] The reason for the haste is unclear, but a royal grant of lands to the abbey may provide a clue. On 7 May 1361, the king granted 'a messuage and a brewhouse called Le Ram' at Tower Hill; other tenements 'which the king had of the grant of Gilbert Bromzerdes, "garlykmongere", and Joan his wife, and Thomas Heywode son and heir of Thomas Heywode … [and] the whole tenement called Le Cornerhouse [also on Tower Hill] … to find chantries and alms in the abbey for the soul of the king and for the soul of his mother Isabel late queen of England'.[380] It may, therefore, be that the king had got wind of a second outbreak as early as March and, through the establishment of chantries in his own royal foundation, was once again keen to improve his spiritual defences.

Royal concern with sanitation and the link between refuse disposal and the plague was once again raised. In May, Edward ordered the removal of slaughterhouses from the city to Stratford or Knightsbridge, complaining to the mayor and commonalty of London that:

> by the killing of great beasts, from whose putrid blood running down the streets and the bowels cast into the Thames, the air in the city is very much corrupted and infected, whence abominable and most filthy stench proceeds, sickness and many other evils have happened to such as have abode in the said city, or have resorted to it; and great dangers are feared to fall out for the time to come, unless remedy be presently made against it.[381]

The wills continue to provide evidence both of the speed of death and the impact the plague had on whole families. Robert de Guldeford, a draper, made his will on 12 May, making provision for his four children. He died within two weeks, and his wife Johanna's will, made on 27 May, specified her burial place by his side in the Lady Chapel of St Augustine Papey. By this time two of their children had also perished, leaving Roesia, 11, and Henry, 9. The remaining two children were placed with different guardians shortly after the enrolment of both parents' wills in December 1361.[382] Nicholas Horewode from the parish of St Nicholas Olave died within two weeks of his will, dated 16 May. In the will he left bequests to his children, but by 7 June, the date of his wife Johanna's will, only one son survived.[383] The number of enrolments in May was eight, matching April's figure, but six of those eight had written their wills since the outbreak of the pestilence.

The crisis once again precipitated confusion among the citizens, exemplified by the family of one victim, Richard de Wycombe. He was a wealthy corder, married with three daughters, one of whom was a nun in Barking Abbey. His will, enrolled on 10 May, made his wife guardian of his youngest daughter, Isabella, and provided for the latter 200 marks of silver for her future marriage and his best silver spice dish. However, by 4 July 1361, it was necessary for the mayor and chamberlain to order the serjeant of the Guildhall to take Isabella, now an orphan, into the city's hands, and to summon the executors of de Wycombe's will. The serjeant reported on the same day that the little girl, said by the executors to be about 9 years old, had been 'carried away' and could not be found; the executors meanwhile brought in the money and the dish to be placed in safekeeping for Isabella's return. The hope of her return was obviously held long, but was ultimately in vain: seven years later, her cousin came to court to claim the legacy, confirming that she had indeed died in 1361.[384] The plague thus probably killed father, mother and at least one daughter.

Some properties, for want of any surviving legal heirs, reverted to the king himself. One example was Edward's grant in fee to John Pecche, a London citizen, of three tenements held by Matilda Wight (died between May and July); and a brewhouse, six shops and a garden at 'Le Barbikan' (in the area of the modern Barbican Centre), which Nicholas de Horewode held (the same Nicholas mentioned above, whose wife also died shortly after). The grant specifically states that 'These all came into the king's hand because the said tenants died without heirs, as has been found by inquisitions',[385] so we may safely assume that de Horewode's son mentioned in his will had also died.

Despite the relatively low enrolment figure, stories such as this hint at how serious an emergency this outbreak was for the city, and soon, as before, it was affecting royal administration. On 10 May the king was compelled to write to Robert de Thorpe, the chief justice, the justices of the Common Bench, and to the treasurer and barons of the Exchequer:

> Whereas great multitudes of the people are suddenly smitten by the deadly plague now newly prevailing both in the City of London and in neighbouring parts, and the plague is daily increasing [in strength], whereby many presenting pleas and business in the king's court have for fear of death drawn to their own parts leaving such pleas and business in peril of loss; wherefore, by assent of the nobles and others of the council, the king has appointed that all pleas pending in the Bench shall be continued [carried forward] in the state they now are until the morrow of mid-summer.[386]

Key personnel in the cathedral and in monastic houses once again fell victim. On the same day as the Common Bench was suspended, the will of William de Ravenstone, the almoner of St Paul's Cathedral – effectively also the schoolmaster – was enrolled. Ravenstone's will, drawn up by him in 1358, is interesting on two counts: first, attached to it was a list of the books of learning he bequeathed to the boys; and second, it provides clear detail of the furnishings and arrangement of the almonry school.[387] The prior of St Bartholomew in Smithfield, John de Carleton, succumbed in early May. On 15 May the king committed to the sub-prior and convent the guardian-ship of the house and all temporalities, 'for as long as it is void following the death of John, the last prior'. The next day, he further provided licence for the sub-prior and convent, 'to elect a prior in the room of John, deceased', and within five days he had signalled his assent to the election of canon Thomas de Watford.[388]

Across the river in Southwark things were no better, and it is probable that plague carried off John de Bradewey, the master of the hospital of St Thomas, before 13 May, when a new master, a former canon from the priory of St Mary Overie called Richard de Stokes, was elected. He, too, was gone before December 1361, the appointment of his successor falling to William Edington as bishop because all the brethren bar one had died in the plague.[389] Secular clergy were no more immune than they had been in the first outbreak, and presentations by the king on 29 May of John de Thorneton, chaplain, to the church of St Dunstan in the West, and on 17 June of Robert de Ellerker, chaplain, to the church of St Stephen Walbrook,[390] suggests losses among the parish incumbents.

In June, will-making peaked at thirty-three, with a quarter of these dating to the three days of the 12th to the 14th. The plague continued to strike rapidly. William Derby, a tailor, made his will on 5 June and was dead and buried at the foot of his father's tomb in the church of St Mary Aldermary by the 12th, when his wife Agnes made her will to be buried at his side under a marble slab.[391] One of the important figures in London's civic administration who drew up wills at this time was Thomas de Walden, former Chamberlain of the Guildhall and principal apothecary of Westminster Abbey since at least 1340. His will was not enrolled until 1362, but his servant and executor, John of Hurley, issued a general release of his role as executor and of Walden's own role as executor to a third party (a cheesemonger called Walter de Blechynglye) to Simon Langham, Abbot of Westminster, on 29 September 1361.[392] Such a release indicates the death of Walden between June and September of that year.

The will of another apothecary, John Offham, was the subject of a remarkable delay in enrolment. Offham, who probably lived in the vicinity of Milk Street, made his will on 16 April and was dead before 26 June, when his son Peter was placed under the guardianship of Thomas Frowyk by the court (Offham's wife and other child, alive in April, were not mentioned so had presumably also perished). The will, however, would wait an astonishing thirty-two years before enrolment in March 1393.[393] An example of a will not enrolled in Husting but which survived in copy form in Chancery was that of William de Neuton, dated 28 June. Probate occurred three weeks later on 19 July. He desired burial in St Stephen Walbrook, leaving money for services for his soul for five years following his death.[394]

One tragic aspect of these wills is the appearance in the Husting rolls of a cluster of fathers wishing to be buried alongside their child or children. Hugh le Peyntor was the most famous of these. He was the same Hugh who had been appointed master painter for the chapel of St Stephen Westminster in March 1350, and was destined to survive until the third outbreak. He nevertheless kept his will dated 16 June 1361, stating his desire to be buried next to his child in the churchyard of St Giles Cripplegate;[395] William Wyle on 20 June chose his burial plot adjacent to the tomb of Alice his daughter in the church of St Sepulchre Newgate; Robert Forneux, a fishmonger, willed burial next to his children in the church of St Leonard Eastcheap (one child survived); and Walter de Chendyngton wished burial next to his children in the churchyard of St Dunstan in the West. The appearance of such cases two months into the plague may indicate that children were among the earlier victims of the outbreak, and may explain why it was considered to have been so virulent among the young. As we will see, the archaeological evidence for the plague's impact on children is less clear-cut than the chroniclers' reports would imply.

Hugh le Peyntor's will, starting with an apt Biblical quote, 'Set thine house in order, for thou shalt die and not live', favoured his local church, St Giles, with bequests to the lights (candles) of the painters, the Holy Trinity, St Mary, and the Fraternity of St George; he also favoured the religious recluses in the vicinity of London and left money to the anchoresses of St Giles, St Benedict and 'St Mary de Manny' (Walter de Mauny's chapel in the West Smithfield plague cemetery); and the hermits of St Lawrence Jewry, Charing Cross, Bishopsgate and 'beyond the Thames'. Le Peyntor's will was not the only one which made bequests to one of London's religious fraternities. A total of thirteen wills made such directions during the plague, equivalent to 10 per cent of all Husting wills drawn up in the plague months, a rate of over six times that in the first plague. If the first plague acted as a catalyst for bequests to these local, craft-based religious groups, then the second outbreak confirmed their importance in the eyes of London's wealthier testators.

Twelve enrolments were made before the court recessed in mid-June; of these ten had been drawn up since the beginning of the plague. One testator, draper Richard atte Moire, whose will was made on 26 April and proved on 14 June, left bequests to both emergency cemeteries at 'Newchurchehawe' and at 'Holy Trinity de la Newchurchehawe near to the Tower',[396] providing important additional confirmation that both the West and East Smithfield cemeteries were still recognised, and were presumably being pressed into use once more for the burial of plague victims. Other wills enrolled in June included Alice de Northall, wife of John, alderman of the city, who had died during the first plague exactly twelve years earlier. Alice chose her burial place by the tomb of her husband in the chapel of St John in the church of St Nicholas Acon.[397]

Of significance also are two wills proved in June which made arrangements to leave money to the 'perpetual chaplains' of St Paul's Cathedral residing in the precinct in a 'common hall' near the dean's mansion.[398] This coincides with a significant increase in will-makers' wishes to be buried at the cathedral during this outbreak, rising in frequency from about 2.5 per cent per annum following the first plague, to over 8 per cent of wills during the *pestis secunda.* An especial focus was the Pardon churchyard there – in June, 12 per cent of will-makers chose that location, and overall, during the second outbreak, fifteen wills (around 11 per cent of the total drawn up) identified it as a preferred burial location. The popularity of this particular churchyard may have been enhanced by an indulgence (as was probably the case in the first plague), the support for the chaplains helping to ensure plentiful intercessory prayers for the souls of the victims and their families.

The plague evidently breached the walls of the Tower of London in June, for the king gave licence for two of his noble French hostages, no less than the son of the French king, Louis, Duke of Anjou, and one Lord Mauleverer:

> [each,] for his health's sake, to go from London, where he is obliged to stay as
> one of the hostages for the performance of the peace with France, to any place
> within the realm for one month from Monday next, on condition that at the
> end of the month he present himself before the king or his council in London,
> as he has promised, to remain a hostage.

One of the knights responsible for the monitoring of the prisoners was Walter de Mauny.[399] The option provided to the French hostages appears to have been a valuable one. John of Byker, the king's master of artillery in the Tower, made his will on 19 June and was dead before 1 July, the day the king granted the office to his son, Patrick, on 12*d* a day (around £18 per annum). John's will was proved three weeks later in the Husting court. Andrew de Turri, the king's smith in the Tower, also perished at about this time. His will is not dated, but in early August the king granted his office to Stephen atte Merssh, 'as much and in such manner as Master Andrew de Turri, late the king's smith took'.[400] A third officer of the Tower may also have succumbed: on 30 August the king issued an arrest warrant for two men who had taken the assets of William de Rothewelle, the keeper of the king's warderobe in the Tower. The latter, in debt to the king, was described as having 'departed this life, and not yet rendered account of such jewels and things'.[401] The plague was still passing through the Tower in September when Sir Thomas of Moray, a Scottish hostage imprisoned since 1357 in the Tower to ensure the repayment of David II of Scotland's ransom, and not apparently given leave of absence, contracted the plague and died there sometime before Michaelmas.[402]

Outside the Tower, another of the king's London servants, John Malewayn, who held the office of 'tronage and pesage' (duties paid for the official weighing of merchandise) of wool imports and exports through London, made his will on 10 June, dying before 28 June. He was buried near his wife in the church of Holy Trinity priory, Aldgate. The king passed the office for life to John Wroth, the Mayor of London.[403] Malewayn may have died at what Italian merchants reported was the peak of the outbreak: the Florentine chronicler Matteo Villani recorded (quite accurately) that the plague had broken out in London in April and (now difficult to prove) that at its peak on 24 June, 1,200 people perished.[404]

Royal favourites were frequently rewarded with corrodies (pensions) within the precincts of particular religious houses. Such people were by no means immune to the pestilence, and at least two corrodians may have died in the priory of St Saviour Bermondsey during the second plague. On 30 June the king sent John Romeseye, one of his esquires, to the prior of Bermondsey, 'to have such maintenance of that house for life as Geoffrey de Sessoun and Colet his wife had', implying that the couple had recently passed away. Another death that occurred there between February and November 1361 was that of William Turk, a citizen and fishmonger favoured by the king since at least the 1330s. In May 1355 a royal grant for life had provided him with a yearly pension of £20 in the priory, a robe of the suit of the priory's esquires, or 20s every Christmas, and two cartloads of good hay yearly from the priory meadows at Bermondsey. The grant itself refers back to a previous royal grant of a house and land within the priory, and we may be sure that Turk lived within the precincts. His will, written and dated 4 February 1361, 'within the cloister' of the priory (named erroneously 'St Mary de Suthwerke'), shows that he enjoyed his pension for over five years. It requested his burial according to the directions of John Asshewell, one of the monks (most likely in the priory church or cemetery), and left the generous sum of 100 marks to the priory.[405]

Such corrodies could be extremely expensive for the host priory, especially given the impact that the plague had on labour and prices. In the face of the death toll, the king's closure of the court of the Common Bench until midsummer proved optimistic, and on 23 June he was forced to extend the closure until September, ordering Robert Thorpe and other justices to adjourn all pleas for Trinity and midsummer in the exact state at which they were 'by reason of the plague both in the City and neighbouring parts'.[406]

July brought no relief from the misery. The national scale of the epidemic is confirmed by the issue of a letter by the Archbishop of York, John Thoresby, dated the 12th of that month. Its content and recommendations for prayers were very similar to instructions issued in 1348, and these were surely spread to Londoners with haste:

> the Kingdom of England has been assailed with ... pestilences and other misfortunes, directed at driving away the sins of men, on such a scale and for such a long time ... Therefore we believe it is important to urge, more devoutly and insistently, suffrages of devout prayer and other offices of pious propitiation.[407]

Thirty-three further wills were drawn up during the month. One such was for the widow Alice Outepenne, daughter of a William de Derby, who desired burial in the Pardon churchyard of St Paul's next to her husband. It may be that her father was the William de Derby buried in St Mary Aldermary less than a month before.[408] Two former mayors also prepared for the worst: Henry Picard, mayor in 1357–8, drew up his will on 3 July, but survived the plague; Richard de Kislingbury was not so lucky and died mid-month. Swifter still was the passing of Richard Lacer, a merchant of Bromley (in Kent) with interests in London. His will was dated 27 July 1361, yet that of his wife Isabella, drawn up just two days later, described her as 'relict of Richard, late mercer'. The gap between death and enrolment was a considerable one – both Lacer wills were enrolled four months later at the end of November.[409]

The plague stalked the halls of the royal palace at Westminster as well as the city streets. On 6 August the king granted to his servant John de Saxton the prebend which John Leche, who died shortly before on 21 July, had in the chapel of St Stephen there.[410] The Husting court, suspended as usual for the Boston fair from 17 June, resumed in late July and a total of thirty-nine wills were enrolled in the two remaining sessions that month. Of these, only four wills had been drawn up before the outbreak of the pestilence and thirty dated to June or July. Given the time-lag between death and enrolment, and the delay for the Boston fair, it is very probable that all these victims died within just a few days of writing their wills. Judging by the rate at which wills were being drawn up and enrolled, the death rate by high summer was comparable with that of January 1349, marking the outbreak as a very serious one indeed.

Despite the availability of the extra-mural plague cemeteries, burial space seems once again to have been an issue. On 26 July the king gave licence for the transfer by Simon de Mordon and his wife Alice to John de Hoghton, parson of the church of St Martin Orgar in Candelwykstrete, of a plot of land in London, 47ft long and 33ft broad (approximately 14m x 10m), situated between St Martin's churchyard and the church of St Michael in Crokedelane, 'for the enlargement of the said churchyard'.[411]

Land transactions and construction by no means ceased during these worst weeks of the outbreak. For example, on 25 June Nicholas, prior of Holy Trinity priory, Aldgate, leased to Nicholas de Donmowe, a carpenter, a tenement with garden in the parish of St Olave by the Tower of London, with a condition that they rebuild the entire street frontage to one storey's height within five years.[412] Many transactions were indeed triggered by plague deaths. William de Preston, one of those who had left money to the common hall of the chaplains at St Paul's, also bequeathed lands in Rotherhithe and Bermondsey to his two sisters, Sarah and Isabella. He died after 24 May, his will being enrolled on 16 June. Three weeks later, on 7 July, his sisters, both now widows, formally granted the land to Thomas Pykenham and Simon Lincoln, citizens, in front of a gathering of several witnesses.[413]

The importance attached to the role of the fraternities in celebrating funerals is clearly set out in the will of one John de Eneveld, penned on 1 April and proved in Husting on 20 July. Leaving a significant property to the fraternity of the Blessed Mary and All Saints in the church of All Hallows by the Wall, of which he was a member, he:

> wills and ordains that the brethren and sisters of his fraternity … attend his funeral at the church of St Audoen, and that born bondmen go to his houses and tenements in Smethfeld after his funeral and there eat together, and by so eating take seisin [possession of the property] for the said fraternity, for which purpose he bequeaths a certain quantity of bread, corn, and malt.[414]

The virulence of the epidemic began to diminish as summer turned to autumn, and will-making dropped to single figures. Only seven wills were drawn up in August, nine in September and six in October, and of this total, four were made by people dwelling in Essex, Middlesex and Kent rather than London. After this period, matters returned to a 'normal' level: collectively the city was no longer in a panic about mortality. The closure of the Husting court for the harvest period of August and September delayed proceedings, and we see a spike in October of twenty-eight enrolments, followed by elevated but diminishing numbers in November (fourteen) and December (eleven).

Among other signs of a return to normal city business was the resumption of the recording of witness of land grants in the City Letter Books.

The earliest which survives is one dated 21 September of a lease by Robert Alyen to John Blake, blader, of a brewery and shops in Thames Street in the parish of St Botolph Billingsgate.[415] Enrolment of October's total complement of twenty-eight wills included just four that had been drawn up before the plague erupted in this year, and only one will that had been written in October itself: the plague had begun to recede. Of the 'plague' wills, sixteen had been made during August and September, when the courts were normally suspended, leading to the large number. Curiously, despite this backlog of work, enrolment of all twenty-eight wills was delayed a further three weeks until the 25th of the month for a reason now unknown. One will proved that day was that of Johanna Hemenhale. She, like Alice de Northall (above), was a plague widow, surviving Edmund Hemenhale, the city sheriff, who had died in the first outbreak. Succumbing in this second pestilence, she left an extensive bequest to found an important chantry in the church of St Martin-le-Grand, and references to this give us the date of her death as 5 September.[416]

By November the plague was clearly faltering. Only two wills were drawn up this month, and of the fourteen enrolled, five had been drawn up well before the plague's outbreak (in one case eighteen years before) and the others were probably remaining backlog. This is demonstrably true for over one-quarter of December's relatively high enrolment total of eleven wills. Among them was that of John Stable, a mercer, whose will dated December 1360 but came to Husting on 13 December 1361. He had died being owed money, and his executors were chasing one debt of £33 15s 6d as early as 1 May. The writ of that date sent to the sheriff of Essex by the Mayor of London described him as 'citizen of London, now deceased'. Robert de Guldeford, already mentioned, had died by 27 May, but his will was enrolled on 10 December; and finally, the Bishop of London, Michael de Northburgh, had died on 9 September, his will being enrolled at the same court as Stable's.[417] We may assume a similar story for many of the others.

The plague appears to have affected the clergy of St Paul's Cathedral significantly. Upon the death of de Northburgh, the king, empowered by the vacancy to appoint officers and to confer prebends, immediately began filling positions. From this we can see that at least six, and possibly as many as nine, former holders of prebends had perished between July and October 1361, out of a total of thirty. These were principally non-resident canons, but significantly, the majority held prebends in proximity to London (such as Hoxton, Wilsden, Mapesbury and Rugmere, near St Pancras). In addition to this, the treasurer and the Archdeacon of Middlesex had both died (as well as the almoner in May). The office for binding the cathedral's books also fell vacant during this time, one William de Mulsho providing the replacement at the king's request.

Other religious houses probably fared no better, but evidence is scant. December saw the appointment of a new master for the hospital of St Thomas in Southwark. The election devolved on the Bishop of Winchester and former treasurer William Edington, 'owing to the death of all the brethren save one'. At the important Hospitaller monastery of St John Clerkenwell, it is significant that in 1361 the number of serving clerks and chaplains at Clerkenwell was well below strength, and at Westminster Abbey the reduction from fifty monks to less than thirty appears to have persisted until the late 1370s. In 1378 the community comprised the abbot and twenty-seven monks, with one more by 1381, though by September 1390 the figure had once again risen to forty-nine monks and the abbot.[418]

The outbreak thus lasted from the middle of April to perhaps the end of October, a total of over six months compared with the nine months of the first main outbreak. It was, therefore, a major event, only eclipsed in the literature and in the records by the magnitude of what had preceded it twelve years earlier. To fully understand the wider impacts on London's population over the century we need to understand better the death toll of this second plague.

Archaeological Evidence for the Pestis Secunda

There is good reason to believe that the East Smithfield cemetery of the Holy Trinity was reused for the burial of some victims of the second pestilence. In March 1350 Edward had presented to the Cistercian order of monks the land adjacent to the cemetery of the Holy Trinity for a new abbey. The cemetery chapel was almost certainly granted to the monks, since in 1351 King Edward made reference to the Royal Free Chapel of the Holy Trinity and of St Mary Graces,[419] but as far as the burial area itself was concerned, the situation is more complex. John Cory, the clerk involved in the cemetery's original foundation, continued his acquisitions and transfer of land to the king for the new abbey, and in August 1353, Edward was able to make a grant:

> [to] the house of St Mary Graces of the Cistercian order, founded by the
> king in the new burial-ground of the Holy Trinity by the Tower of London,
> of all the toft and place of land newly dedicated for the said burial-ground
> and all the messuages, houses, garden, curtilage and lands at Estsmethfeld and

la Tourhull … which tenements John Cory granted to the king in fee, to augment the endowment already made them by the king of messuages at la Tourhull which he likewise had of the grant of the said John.[420]

By 1353, the Cistercians owned the land. However, the cemetery remained as a separate entity in the minds of Londoners until at least 1361. In December 1351 Johanna Cros made bequests to the 'new sepulchre of Blessed Virgin without Aldersgate' and to the 'like work of the Holy Trinity towards the Tower'; and in 1361 Richard de Moire's will likewise specified 'Holy Trinity de la Newchurchehawe near the Tower'. The fact that the monks built their first, small cloister to the south of the chapel, away from the cemetery, despite the relatively confined space available,[421] suggests that they too were respecting this entity. The answer to this lies in the fact that the land occupied by the cemetery had been passed to the abbey, but rights of burial and the income resulting, held by the prior of Holy Trinity Aldgate, had not. The latter were, in fact, held by the prior until 1364, when Simon, Bishop of London, ruled that 'oblations arising from the cemetery newly consecrated close to the Tower … shall be converted [from Holy Trinity priory] to the use of the abbey of St Marys Graces'. Thus, during the second plague, the cemetery was directly adjacent to, but remained administratively separate from, the new abbey.

The confusion in the popular eye caused by this odd situation is neatly captured by Richard de Walsted's will of July 1365, leaving money to the 'abbey of Holy Trinity near Towrhille'.[422] The cemetery was still available for burial without recourse to the new abbey, the rights of burial residing with Holy Trinity priory as they had during the first outbreak. After 1364, the monks owned and managed the land outright, and no further surviving wills make reference to the cemetery of the Holy Trinity. It is believed that the plague cemetery area was no longer physically available for burial by 1405, since a tenement belonging to William and Katherine Somers existed by that date to the north of the Great Court and abbey church door (and thus in the area of the plague cemetery), and included a garden that took in part of the abbey churchyard.[423] This provides us with a 'latest date' for any burials made following the 1349 outbreak.

Archaeologically, burials encountered on the site of the cemetery and abbey split into three principal groups: those which certainly dated to the 1349 outbreak, already discussed; a later group of 228 graves lying above the western 1349 cemetery plot and in many cases cutting into the mass trenches and individual graves; and a group of ninety-seven burials lying in a separate space between the western and eastern 1349 plots, centred on a

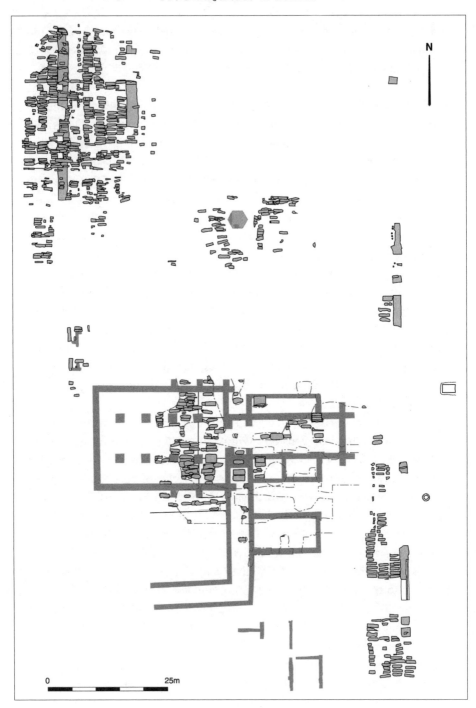

Fig. 14 The archaeological evidence for the East Smithfield cemetery and the later abbey and churchyard of St Mary Graces, founded 1353 (compare with Fig. 4). (Courtesy of Museum of London Archaeology)

stone churchyard cross base (see Fig. 14). It is the group of 228 overlying the 1349 cemetery, previously considered to have belonged to the abbey cemetery, which were most probably buried in the *pestis secunda*.

The features which suggest this interpretation are physical location, archaeological dating evidence and, most suggestive of all, the similarity of demographic make-up and burial practice between the group and the earlier, underlying burials from the first outbreak. This area of burial was at a significant distance from the site of the abbey church – the nearest known burial from the group was over 30m to the north of the church. A separate burial area (of ninety-seven graves) which most certainly did function as the abbey cemetery lay 12m to the east of the group. It lay in the land which had been unused at the time of the first plague, and was centred on a churchyard cross. The group has the appearance of a completely separate entity.

The archaeological dating evidence from the group of 228 graves is very slender. In the absence of any radiocarbon dating, the only burial which could be dated was that of a man buried clothed: a pair of breche buckles was recovered from the grave, and these are fairly securely dated to no later than *c.* 1400. Dating evidence from the adjacent abbey cemetery was equally thin, but what we do have suggests a later period: an adult whose bones have been radiocarbon-dated to 1402–1625;[424] and an older man buried with a shoe buckle which is thought to be of fifteenth-century date. The proposed chronology of the area of the plague cemetery is not refuted by the evidence. However, it is the nature of the people buried there and how they were buried which provides the sharpest contrast between this group and those clustered around the abbey cross. First, the demography shows marked differences. The proportion of children in the latter was much lower – 17 per cent of the total as compared with nearly 33 per cent in the group overlying the plague cemetery. The number of women around the cross was also lower – 25 per cent compared with 40 per cent in the plague cemetery area. And, as Table 4a shows, where age and sex can be compared together, those buried around the cross were likely to have been significantly older at the time of death – one in four were in their forties, compared to one in eleven in the plague cemetery. The group of 228 are, therefore, simultaneously very different from those buried around the abbey cross and very similar to those buried in the earlier plague cemetery.

This comparison is reinforced when the use of coffins for burial is examined. Coffins were used to bury nearly 49 per cent of all the dead found on the plague cemetery site, a close comparison with the figure for the individual graves from the 1349 plague, but very much greater than the figure of 23 per cent for those buried around the cross. Taking a wider, national

Age	1361	1349	Abbey	Age	1361	1349	Abbey	Age	1361	1349	Abbey
Young men	9%	14%	13%	Mature men	43%	48%	46%	Old men	8%	5%	15%
Young women	9%	6%	5%	Mature women	27%	24%	10%	Old women	3%	4%	10%

Table 4a. Proportions of the adult population of all burials where both an age and a sex could be established for the 1361 burials, compared with the 1349 group and those buried around the abbey churchyard cross.

Infants	12%		
Children/teens	23%		
Young men	6%	Young women	6%
Mature men	28%	Mature women	18%
Old men	5%	Old women	2%

Table 4b. Age and sex distribution of the skeletons buried in the East Smithfield cemetery, probably in the pestis secunda of 1361.

perspective, the demographic and cultural pattern displayed by the plague cemetery groups (both that of 1349 and the later group) is dissimilar to any other published cemetery to date, while the general structure of the group from around the churchyard cross is repeated at a number of monastic sites.[425]

In aggregate, the historical and archaeological evidence combines to reinforce the notion that the group buried on the 1349 plague plot was indeed formed principally of victims of the second plague. If this is correct, then we can make some very tentative observations about the differences between the two plague groups. The overall nature of the cemetery population, using the same recorded data as for 1349, is very similar. The number of infant deaths is slightly greater, that of teens a little less, and the overall proportions buried suggests that the 1361 outbreak was only very slightly more dangerous to the young than that of 1349. This may not be so surprising since the majority of the youngsters represented in this group would have been born after 1349, and so would possess no immunity (unless any were transmitted from mothers who had survived).

In conclusion, the East Smithfield cemetery appears to have been reused for plague burials as one of two cemeteries specifically set up in 1349 for dealing with the crisis; the burials indicate that the second outbreak was of a very similar nature to the first in terms of the population; and the burial customs employed were also very similar.

The Effects of the Pestis Secunda

Such consideration as has been given to the direct impacts of the 1361 outbreak in the literature has mainly attempted to provide a national picture, suggesting a mortality of between 4.5 to 6 times the average for the first half of the fourteenth century,[426] suggesting that the outbreak was up to one-third as powerful as the 1349 pestilence. In London itself previous estimates suggest that things were worse, perhaps as much as nine times the average death rate of the ten years since 1351.[427] However, a closer look at the evidence from the enrolments, taking into account the already reduced population, suggests an even higher mortality. A total of ninety-five wills were enrolled in the seven months between the beginning of April and the end of October 1361. This compares to a minimum of 135 wills enrolled between April 1351 and March 1361, a figure that should be increased (by around ten) to account for the missing enrolments of 1360. This actually represents a factor of over eleven times the annual rate of this decade, a disaster of major proportions. Certainly, Parliament raised the issue of the labour laws and of the prices for employing clergy once more, and both the king and the lords spiritual responded by restricting wages and stipends as they had in 1349–51.

The signs are that fertility rates were down and mortality rates up in the aftermath of the first outbreak, but our only clue as to the extent to which London had repopulated itself before the *pestis secunda* is the 1357 description of the city as one-third empty. This is obviously a very crude indicator, but we should anticipate a slow recovery, mainly through immigration. Reproductive recovery rates appear to have been severely reduced. Allowing an entirely nominal 2 per cent net increase each year after 1349 (the equivalent of two people arriving per day), the population would recover from *c.* 33,000 after the first outbreak to perhaps 42,000 by 1361. The estimate of mortality in the second plague would reduce such a figure to as few as 34,000 in the space of six months or so.

There is little direct London evidence for the chroniclers' claims that the second outbreak attacked children in greater numbers than the first. One indirect indicator may be the appearance in the Husting wills of testators' preference for burial near the tombs or graves of their predeceased offspring. As noted above, four wills were made with this specification, all during the pestilence, and all were made two months or more after the beginning of the outbreak. Of course, we do not know how old these four testators were, or when their children died, but cluster (4 per cent of wills made during the plague months) is probably significant; there was just one example from among all the wills enrolled during the 1348–9 outbreak.[428]

The restriction of these wills to the last two months of the plague may indeed support reports in the chronicles that the second plague affected children first, and adults later. It seems more likely to this author that the belief that the second plague disproportionately affected the young arose through the value parents and families attached to the post-1350 generation and younger survivors of the first outbreak – it would have seemed so much more dangerous to them. In support of this, the use of coffins for infants and children at the East Smithfield cemetery increased dramatically from 20 per cent in the 1348–9 outbreak to over 51 per cent in the *pestis secunda*. If this was representative of child deaths across the city, the effort of preparation for the burial of children was clearly much greater than in the first plague.

The remarkable thing about the second pestilence is that it was a major disaster on its own terms. Approximately 34 per cent of London's population died. If the 1349 plague had not occurred, it is probable that the impact of such an outbreak would have featured prominently in historical analyses of the fourteenth century. Like an aftershock to a massive earthquake, it is seldom reported on in detail, but its effects must surely have amplified considerably the enormous damage wreaked by the first plague. And, like an aftershock, it was to be followed just seven years later by a third visitation.

The Third Plague, 1368

There is some confusion over the date of the third outbreak. The Anonimalle Chronicle (written at the abbey of St Mary, York) noted that 'in 1369 there was a third pestilence in England and in several other countries. It was great beyond measure, lasted a long time and was particularly fatal to children.' The Chronicle of the Greyfriars of King's Lynn also repeats 1369 as the year in which 'there occurred a great pestilence of nobles and children'.[429] Indeed, many principal commentators since have noted that the plague was confined to that year.[430] However, a chronicle of Peterborough Abbey describes how in the third pestilence in 1368, among the dead were a great number of foreigners in London.[431] The evidence from both the Husting wills and the wills proved in the Archdeaconry Court of London are categorical in demonstrating that the plague affected the south of the country from about May 1368, probably fading out in the city around October of that year.

While the Archdeaconry Court testaments do not survive before 1393, an index of those from 1368 does,[432] and analysis of this shows that 180 records of will and/or probate were registered between May and October 1368, over three times the average non-plague yearly figure of just under sixty probates in that court.[433] There was an overlap between those whose wills were proved in the Archdeaconry Court and those, owning estate in the city, who wished subsequently to have wills enrolled in Husting. However, the relationship is complex. First, the jurisdiction of the Archdeaconry Court covered only about half the city parishes, but included some of the larger extra-mural parishes such as St Leonard Shoreditch and St Mary Clerkenwell. Second, not everyone who could have their will proved at the Archdeaconry Court either wished to or could also afford to have it enrolled in the Husting court. Third, not everyone who owned estate in the city dwelled in the jurisdiction of the archdeacon. Thus, of 193 testamentary records dating to 1368, just thirteen (6.7 per cent) were written by individuals who also paid for Husting will enrolments. Conversely, those who had their wills proved at the Archdeaconry Court made up a significant 46 per cent of all Husting enrolments for 1368. The link between the two courts provides further evidence of the potential lag between probate and subsequent enrolment at Husting. Of the thirteen Husting wills, seven were enrolled after the summer fair recess of August and September, all on 16 October 1368, but the remaining six wills took up to a year after this date to appear on the Husting rolls. Of these, three could have been plague victims since their wills were drawn up during the plague months. Extrapolated, this suggests that of the twenty-eight wills enrolled later, during 1369, seven were probably proved as a result of plague death, bringing the total to thirty-five.

The twenty-eight wills enrolled at Husting in 1368 provide some flavour of the march of the epidemic. The outbreak probably began in late April or early May, shown by the evidence of two new wills drawn up in the last week of April and another seven by the end of May. Prior to this, only three wills had been drawn up in the previous five months. Of these nine, two willed burial in the churchyard of St Paul's – one, the goldsmith John Hiltoft, specifying the Pardon churchyard. The other, Henry Yerdelee, left a bequest for a chantry to be founded in the chapel of the Holy Trinity at the 'new cemetery towards the Tower', the plague cemetery at East Smithfield. A third, carpenter Robert de Watford, specified the 'Pardonchirchehawe' of St Bartholomew's priory, almost certainly de Mauny's adjacent West Smithfield foundation, or possibly a cemetery by that name within the precincts of the priory itself.[434] In this small sample, then, there is good evidence of themes common to previous outbreaks.

The plague was evidently of sufficient severity for Edward to completely suspend the business of the King's Bench, Common Pleas and the upper Exchequer on 22 May until 30 September; the exchequer of receipt, also based in Westminster Palace, did stay open but conducted business on only three days during this period, a consequence and illustration of the impact the plague had on economic activity.[435] Significantly, the king had pressed ahead with his Parliament at Westminster between 1 and 21 May, indicating either that the business to be discussed was of too great importance to be delayed, or that the pestilence was not considered to be as potent as in previous outbreaks. It may have been the latter, for in the city the Husting and other courts continued to be held throughout the outbreak, unlike on previous occasions. The Letter Books and the Pleas and Memoranda rolls both show activity throughout the plague, with records set down from April through to August, and the Assize of Nuisance held throughout April, May and June (though there was a pause between 30 June and 21 October).[436]

Amidst this activity are the inevitable guardianship hearings for children orphaned from the death of their father or of both parents. The earliest example during the outbreak was held on 4 May and concerned Alice, 7-year-old daughter of Nicholas de Pekham.[437] Alice appeared in a custody hearing just a month later, since one of the relatives to whom she had been assigned had by then himself died. Other similar cases highlight probable plague deaths. Orphan Johanna, aged 8, daughter of Walter de Harwedone, was committed to William de Harwedone, her uncle, on 13 July. Sureties for her were paid by three men, including one Thomas Wylby who himself succumbed that year; his will was proved by the Archdeaconry Court within two months of the hearing.[438] Draper Thomas de Welforde had died during the 1361 outbreak, leaving his estate to his wife Johanna and his children John, Elizabeth and Johanna. Between his death and 1368, both John and Elizabeth also died, leaving the last child, Johanna, the sole beneficiary under the guardianship of a Michael Ede. On 3 July 1368 Michael brought Johanna to the Guildhall handing her and her property into trust. Three weeks later, she was committed to a new guardian, draper Richard de Kyllyngworth, but within a few weeks she perished.[439]

Two unusual and linked cases were heard in court on 19 June, each passing custody of three children to their respective, and still living, fathers, William de Tyngewyk and Henry de Markeby. Children who still had a father did not come under the jurisdiction of the mayor and aldermen, and it seems that in these cases the children had received a bequest from the will of a third party, the mechanism of guardianship being used to protect that inheritance from waste through the process of providing sureties. Both men were goldsmiths, and this, coupled with the fact that both of the assignments of guardianship happened on the same day, suggests the bequest came from another goldsmith.[440]

June was, curiously, unremarkable in terms of wills: just four were drawn up and one enrolled – figures which would not in themselves suggest plague.

However, corroborative evidence from another town, Derby, makes it clear that much of England was in the grip of the disease by this time. On 12 June Edward issued royal protection for the town, its burgesses and merchants, because it was:

> for the most part wasted by the death of burgesses and other men of the town in the present pestilence, and the men now remaining are not sufficient to maintain and govern the town, and that the men of the adjacent country, whom they cannot resist, depasture and tread down the said pastures with their animals.[441]

July was rather different. Ten wills were drawn up, eight of them in the last week of the month, suggesting that conditions were especially grim. Of these, one was for John Lovekyn, the man whose mayoralty had spanned the first great outbreak and who had gone on to be mayor three more times until his death some time before November 1368. Another was for chandler William Hathefeld, whose testament was proved in the Archdeaconry Court in 1368, before being enrolled at Husting in January 1369.[442] Other wills did exist which were neither listed in the Archdeaconry Court registers nor in Husting, such as that of Robert Faukes of Gaddesby, tailor and citizen of London, dated 18 July. He requested burial in Holy Trinity priory beside Robert, his uncle, and left 20*s* to the box of the tailors' fraternity of his trade, along with cloth to be sold and the proceeds distributed to the poor.[443] Wills of non-residents (proved in courts outside London) make it clear that many who lived beyond the city walls had significant interests in London, and indeed probably died there (not necessarily of plague it should be noted). One such was Robert de Pleseleye, rector of the church of Southfleet, in the diocese of Rochester. His will, dated at London on 22 May 1368, 'in my dwelling [*hospicio*] in St Martin le Grand Lane', and proved on 7 August, set out his desire to be buried in the church of St Martin-le-Grand, and left over £13 to the friaries and nunneries of the city.[444]

The summer progression of the pestilence raised once again the perceived dangers surrounding animal slaughter and butchery in and around the city. On 3 July the mayor, Simon de Mordon, and his aldermen, received a writ from Edward III enclosing the complaint from no less than the Bishop of London, the Earls of Warwick and Salisbury, the Countess of Pembroke, and other residents of Old Dean's Lane alleging that the butchers of the Shambles (near Greyfriars):

who used to slaughter their cattle and leave their offal and refuse outside the City, had recently taken to slaughtering … within the City, carrying the offal and offensive refuse by day and night through Oldedeneslane and by the King's Wardrobe to a small plot by the Thames close to the Friars Preachers, to the grievous corruption of the water.

The writ demanded that the practice be stopped. The mayor initiated an inquest covering four wards – Castle Baynard, Farringdon Without, Vintry and Queenhithe – to discover the extent of the problem of disposing offal and waste in the Thames, and the extent to which people considered it a real nuisance. A jury of twelve men from Castle Baynard ward found that it was indeed the Shambles butchers who carted their offal to a place called Butchers Bridge ('Bochersbregge'), near Baynard Castle, and not only was it polluting the river, but blood from slaughter yards and offal dropped from carts fouled the streets and lanes, too. It was recommended that slaughter should take place beyond the city walls.[445]

Will-making in August was still at an elevated rate. Thirteen such wills were later enrolled in Husting. Among them was that of William de Burton, a goldsmith, who drew up his will on 31 August. His wife and executrix was disposing of property to third parties within four weeks of this date, so we may be confident that he had passed away within a week or two of making his will. Pepperer John de Evenefeld included in his will a rather curious stipulation: 'his body not to be left above ground, but to be placed in a chest [coffin] underground, and to be previously covered with 10 ells of black or russet cloth'. Why he wished this treatment, and how it might have differed from a standard funeral, is not clear, but it suggests that he did not wish a period of watch or wake over his body either at his home or in church.[446] He willed burial in the church of St Mary Aldermary, next to his first wife. Burial space appears not to have been the issue it had been during the earlier outbreaks, despite the fact that the emergency cemetery at East Smithfield had certainly gone out of use by this time. There is a reference to the enlargement of the cemetery of St Leonard Eastcheap in this year,[447] but this seems a somewhat piecemeal response and rather underscores the sense that this pestilence was less severe than previous outbreaks.

The beginning of the end of the outbreak came in September. Only four wills were drawn up, in one of which John Briklesworth requested burial in the Pardon churchyard at St Paul's. As with August, the intermission of the Husting court for the harvest meant that no enrolments took place. These were left over until October (or later), in which month just three wills were drawn up, returning the level of will-making to a pre-plague scale. Two of these wills are significant. The first, apparently a nuncupative will given on 29 October, is the only will in the entire Husting roll which mentions pestilence. It is that of an Ipswich man with commercial property in the city:

> In the name of God, amen. I, Richard of Holewelle of Ipswich, being of sound mind and good memory, seeing the danger of this world and especially of this pestilence, establish my will for my freehold in the city of London in this form. First I leave all this holding with three shops adjoining and all things pertaining to them … to Geoffrey Sterling, Robert of Preston and John Holt of Ipswich and their heirs and assigns, to have and to hold in perpetuity. In witness of this, I have affixed my seal, and because my seal is unknown to many, I have arranged for the seal of the office of the bailiffs of the town of Ipswich to be affixed.[448]

The second will of importance is that dated 14 October, of Simon Benyngton, a draper. He bequeathed a quitrent for the maintenance of a chantry at the altar of St Mary in Gysma (in childbirth), probably situated in the Lady Chapel in the priory of St Thomas Acon. This is the earliest reference to such an altar, and its dedication in the face of successive child-killing plagues is likely to have carried a particular resonance. Benyngton's will was enrolled in December, but he was certainly dead by the beginning of November.[449]

The backlog of enrolments brought the total for October to sixteen. Of these, thirteen were enrolled on one day (16 October). Only one of these had been penned before the outbreak of the plague, making it very likely that the majority of the remainder were victims of the disease. Among them were John Deynes (who had died before 1 September) and his son Henry. The latter, choosing not to pass his inheritance on to his stepmother, John's second wife, instead bequeathed the proceeds to the maintenance of a clock on the church of St Pancras, a new belfry at St Margaret Lothbury, and the maintenance of six Oxford scholars. Such were the winners and losers during the epidemic. November and December saw further enrolments of wills of those who had died in the outbreak, but in smaller numbers. It is clear that by the end of October, the pestilence had once again passed.

The impact of the third plague is hard to gauge. Wills enrolled at Husting averaged sixteen annually between 1362 and 1367; the total number likely to have been associated with the seven plague months, enrolled in 1368 and 1369, was thirty-five – a figure 3.8 times higher. An annual average of eight Husting wills were drawn up over the same six-year period; in the seven pestilence months of April to October that figure was forty-four, eight times higher. On the face of it, this suggests a mortality of about 11 per cent, but an expectation of mortality that was far greater. Even if we allow again for an (unproven) increase of 2 per cent per annum in the resident population of London from 34,000 in 1361 to 39,000 by 1368, this suggests that the population fell again to perhaps 35,000 by the winter of that year.

The constant erosion of London's population must have had a significant long-term impact on a wide range of institutions in the city. There is little direct evidence of this, although problems of recruitment at two religious houses in 1370–1 may be represented by the fact that four acolytes were ordained as canons for the hospital of St Mary within Cripplegate (Elsyng Spital) in St Paul's Cathedral on 21 December 1370; and in October 1371 Raymond Berengar, master of the entire order of Hospitallers, was forced to write to John Dalton, the prior of the church of St John Clerkenwell, ordering him to restore the number of chaplains serving in the church from around seven to the appointed fifteen.[450] So, 1368 appears to have been considerably less severe than either of the two previous outbreaks, but was nonetheless a notable event in its own right, perhaps killing upwards of 4,000 of London's pestilence-weary population.

The Fourth Plague, 1375

In 1374 the fourth pestilence began in England in several towns in the south of the country. In the following year a large number of Londoners, from among the wealthier and more eminent citizens, died in the pestilence. Several well-placed clerks of the Chancery, Common Pleas and Exchequer also died.

In 1375 the weather was scorching and there was a great pestilence which raged so strongly in England and elsewhere that infinite numbers of men and women were devoured by sudden death.[451]

The last plague under consideration in this volume broke out in London towards the end of May 1375, persisting across the summer months until about the middle of August.[452] Just two wills enrolled in Husting were made in the second half of May, one by carpenter Richard de Chelmeresford and one by vintner John de Rothyng, and while this presents no evidence for the plague's outbreak, de Rothyng's will dated 23 May is interesting. In it he specified that the bodies of his father Richard and mother Salerna should be exhumed from where they lay and placed with him in his chosen burial place in the floor at the centre of the belfry of St James Garlickhythe, a definitive example of the increasing interest in co-locating family burial.

The number of enrolments in May was also normal and probably unrelated to plague deaths. One was that of Adam Fraunceys, the influential mercer who had been alderman and then mayor in the 1350s. By it, he set up two chantry chapels in the Benedictine nunnery of St Helen's Bishopsgate, one dedicated to the Blessed Virgin and the other to the Holy Ghost; he also bequeathed money for the marriage portions of unmarried poor girls, a facet of late fourteenth-century will-making to which we shall return in the concluding chapter.[453]

This was a slow start, and the outbreak gathered speed only in the latter half of June. Twelve wills were made of which seven occur in the last ten days of the month.[454] The will of William Olneye, fishmonger, drawn up on 24 June, was careful to specify the place of his burial in the church of St Mary at Hill, 'before the Salutation of the Blessed Virgin Mary where Salve is daily sung'; such a location was quite possibly triggered by a desire for the Virgin's intercession during plague.[455] Dramatic evidence of sudden death and rapid remarriage among families is provided through the Pleas and Memoranda rolls from January 1376. In January 1375 Adam Cope, a skinner, drew up his will leaving his estate to his wife Agnes and their five children, John, William, Joan, Alice and Maud. Three of the children, William, Alice and Maud, perished on a single day (18 June), Adam himself having already died. The mother remarried four days later and, it was alleged, with her new husband, dispossessed her own son John from a tenement and shops he believed were his.[456]

July saw a further increase in the rate at which wills were being drawn up. A combined total of thirty-eight survive in the indexes of the Archdeaconry and Commissary Courts, and in the Husting rolls.[457] Of thirty-four in the court indexes, ten (29 per cent) were subsequently enrolled at Husting. The total of Husting enrolments made in June was thirteen, of which these ten represent 77 per cent: therefore, most of the Husting wills were enrolled by Londoners. Notable among them were William Herland, the king's chief carpenter in the 1350s and responsible for major work at Windsor, the Tower of London and Westminster Abbey. He was dead within ten days of making his will and was buried in his local parish church of St Peter Paul's Wharf, 'before the image of St Katherine' in the Lady Chapel there. John de Mitford, a draper, left in his will money to the rector and his fellow parishioners of St Mary Magdalen Milk Street for the good of his family's souls, but with a note stating that if his bequest was in some manner illegal, then the rightful heirs should use the money for the same purpose. This suggests that it was difficult if not impossible for de Mitford to establish the proper checks himself.[458]

Of the makers of the thirteen Husting wills dated in July, four were dead before the month was out. A total of seven wills were enrolled during July. Also dead was the long-standing master of the hospital of St James near Westminster, John de Norwich. His will was proved in the Commissary Court before 30 July, the date his replacement Thomas de Orgrave was recognised. John de Norwich was the (until now unrecognised) head of the hospital, running it from at least 1354.[459] Apostasy from religious houses may have been at least partly responsible for the issue on 20 July by the king of an order 'to all sheriffs and bailiffs to arrest all those of the order of Friars Preachers whom they shall find vagabond in their bailiwicks, as the prior provincial or any prior conventual of the said order shall intimate to them, and to deliver them to the said priors'.[460]

The seriousness of the plague was confirmed on 15 July when Simon Sudbury, Archbishop of Canterbury, sent out a letter requesting penitential processions, using the following words:

> Would that those ... who give their attention to the mortality, pestilence or epidemic now reigning in England ... could be persuaded to pour out unceasing prayers to the most high for the cessation of this pestilence or epidemic ... in our modern times we are mired in monstrous sin and the lack of devotion among the people provokes the great king to whom we should direct our prayers. As a result we are assailed by plagues or epidemics.[461]

The weather during the summer raised another spectre – that of fire in the city. The temperature soared and at the end of the month the mayor ordered the aldermen to see that in front of every house in each ward 'there should stand a large cask or other vessel full of water during the presently intense hot and dry season, that there should be ladders and crooks, and that the watches should be properly kept'.[462] The existence of this precautionary edict is interesting insofar as it contrasts with any direct reference to the pestilence itself. It is a reminder, perhaps, of the difference between positive action to ward off a risk that was physical and preventable and the lack of any coherent response to an intangible punishment brought down by a wrathful God.

Eight Husting wills were drawn up in August, six in the first fortnight. All except one came before the Archdeaconry (four) or Commissary Courts for probate. They included the will of skinner Henry de Sudbury, a man clearly very keen on religious houses. His two sons, John and William, were monks at Battle Abbey and Westminster, while his daughter Agnes was a nun at the Franciscan convent of St Clare in the Minories;[463] he also left the bed 'where he may die' to a sister in the hospital of St Katherine by the Tower. His probate is dated to 1375, but it took until 1381 for his will to be enrolled in Husting. Across two ecclesiastical courts, probate of eighteen separate wills took place in August,[464] but no details of enrolments exist since the Husting court was closed for August and September.

August raised once again fears about lepers and leprosy, and the keepers of the city gates, including those of London Bridge and the Tower postern gate, were instructed not to allow lepers to enter the city. The instructions were explicit. They were to prohibit lepers from the city and suburbs, restraining them if necessary, and failure would be met with a grim punishment:

> that they will well and trustily keep the Gates and Postern aforesaid ... and will not allow lepers to enter the City, or to stay in the same, or in the suburbs thereof; and ... if any lepers or leper shall come there, and wish to enter, such persons or person shall be prohibited by the porter from entering; and if, such prohibition notwithstanding, such persons or person shall attempt to enter, then they or he shall be distrained by their or his horses or horse, if they or he shall have any such, and by their outer garment ... And if even then such persons or person shall attempt to enter, they or he shall ... in safe custody be kept ... And further, the same porters were told, on pain of the pillory, that they must well and trustily observe and keep this Ordinance, as aforesaid.[465]

The strategy was extended in the same instruction to attempt to cut off any possible contamination at source: the 'foremen' of the leper hospitals of the Lock in Southwark and Hackney, just north of the city, were also required to swear that 'they will not bring lepers, or know of their being brought, into the City aforesaid; but that they will inform the said porters, and prevent the said lepers from entering, so far as they may'. Leprosy was, of course, feared generally, but this order, examined in the light of the concerns over roaming lepers from St Giles in 1354, raises the possibility that outbreaks of plague may have hardened the hearts of civic authorities against a somewhat laxer approach normally taken towards London's lepers. The issue of lepers is touched upon further in the concluding chapter.

Following the harvest recess, the Husting court reconvened on 15 October, and again one week later. It enrolled twelve wills, the earliest of which dated to late June and the latest to 6 September. These, and one or two in November, represented the rather modest tail end of the fourth plague, the last outbreak to blight Edward III's reign.

The impact of this plague was undoubtedly much less than that of those preceding it. Overall, 237 wills were proved in London's ecclesiastical courts during the whole year of 1375. Of the thirty-six wills enrolled in Husting, eighteen were from this probate number, leaving an equal number of wills probably proved outside London courts. To this number we can add the cases of those who had died intestate, also the responsibility of the courts. The complexities surrounding claims against such estates meant that there was a lag in hearings and judgements, so the numbers extend well beyond the end of the outbreak. Sixteen such cases occurred in 1375, twenty-five in 1376, and twenty-three in the final year of Edward's reign.[466] The level of mortality associated with the pestilence itself is as ever difficult to calculate, but we do have two wills series to compare.

The average number of Husting enrolments between 1370 and 1374 was fourteen per annum, or about 3.5 every three months. A total of twenty-three wills were enrolled during or as a direct result of the three plague months, an additional mortality of 5.4 times the normal figure. The Archdeaconry Court figures suggest something a little lower than this. The average annual probate rate for the same five-year period between the third and fourth plagues was fifty-eight wills. This equates to an additional mortality level during the three months of about 4.1 times the pre-outbreak figure. We should, therefore, work on an estimated mortality rate about five times greater than in the years since the third plague. The duration is critical here – only just three months. It is this which saved the city from another terrible hammering, as the death toll may have been as low as 1,500 in this outbreak, or nearly 4 per cent of the population. London in 1375 may, therefore, have had as few as 38,000 residents.

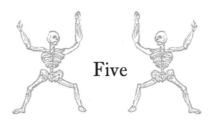

Five

SOCIAL CONSEQUENCES
OF THE PLAGUE

PLAGUE OUTBREAKS in London continued well past the period of this study, throughout the fifteenth century and beyond, and the first four epidemics of pestilence in particular, all occurring within a twenty-eight-year period, cannot but have had significant effects on the behaviour and lifestyle of London's residents. However, the first outbreak arrived at a time of significant change and upheaval – a generation earlier England had experienced a significant and prolonged famine, while wars with France and Scotland ran a parallel track with the disease. In addition, important cultural changes in architecture, ceramics and textiles were already under way before 1348. As many historians have been at pains to point out, it is extremely hard, therefore, to differentiate between changes in the late fourteenth century which would have arrived in any event, from those that were catalysed, accelerated or shaped by the experience of four epidemics and, finally, from those changes which could be laid squarely at the door of the disease itself. This chapter builds on the immediate impacts identified in Chapter 3 and sets out some broader aspects of change in later fourteenth-century London which appear to be related, sometimes quite clearly, to the advent of the plague and which may deserve closer scrutiny.

The most obvious change in London was that there were far fewer people by the end of the century than there had been in 1348. London lost perhaps 55–60 per cent of its population in the first outbreak. The critical information – the gross rate of replacement – is unclear, and will probably elude any accurate calculation. However, the estimates from the will rates presented in earlier chapters allow some basis for the rather more robust figures included in the Poll Tax of 1377. For this tax, a total of 23,314 lay persons over 14 years of age were assessed in London. This figure did not include children under 14, homeless paupers, clergy or aliens. We know that avoidance was likely and that this figure is likely to have been a considerable underestimate. Over the river in Southwark, the 1381 Poll Tax assessed 1,060 individuals, calculated to represent up to 2,100 residents, inclusive of paupers, children, aliens and clergy. In Westminster, the 1377 Poll Tax assessed 280 persons but it has been shown that the more likely population for the vill by the end of the century was around 2,000, and that inward migration and growth cannot have been the cause. In London itself, the assessed figures have been suggested to represent 35,000 residents, assuming that 30 per cent of the total adult population was under 14.[467] A figure of 40 per cent is now more commonly applied to the cohort under 14 years of age, which would give a number of about 39,000 inhabitants.

Such figures are broadly consistent with suggestions made above about the mortality rates from each pestilence outbreak and subsequent population recovery. In the absence of any more detailed information, we can suggest that the net reduction in population was in the region of 40–45 per cent between 1348 and 1380. Accepting this figure, it seems unquestionable that the character of the city changed dramatically. It was now nearly half-empty of residents, if not necessarily of visitors, even though it had probably been topped up by inward migration throughout the decades as newcomers sought to take advantage of the opportunities. Such migration can be seen in the fact that as many as 65 per cent of grocers' guild members listed in 1373 had no previous known connection with the trade in the city and many seemed to be new to London entirely.[468]

The composition of this reduced population may also have changed. Using evidence from the London Court of Orphans, it has been calculated that the average sex ratio (males to females) was 1.33:1 between 1309 and 1348. This figure dropped to 1.17:1 from 1349 to 1398. A more detailed consideration of the period 1375–99 suggests a ratio of 1.12:1. This can be considered in the light of evidence from the Husting wills. As seen above (Chapter 3) for the decade from August 1349 to July 1359, the sex ratio of children mentioned in the Husting wills was 1.27:1, dropping to 1.22:1 for the period August 1349 to December 1375. On the face of it, the numbers of men and women were becoming more equal. The London tax return for 1377 suggests a ratio of 1.07:1, and work on other towns in England indicate even lower ratios by 1381, including Southwark at 1.02:1. It has been suggested that this phenomenon is partly related to an increase in female migration from rural districts to the town.[469]

The overall demographic shrinkage should have affected the physical structure of the city, but clear evidence is lacking. We know that in 1357 Londoners (trying to reduce their royal taxation burden) were claiming that one-third of the city's buildings lay vacant. While this may have been exaggerated, it cannot have been implausible since the city's proximity to the royal palace at Westminster meant that the king's agents could easily investigate the matter for themselves. The better trading or craft zones may have been able to capitalise on this, attracting inward migration at the expense of poorer or more marginal districts. A study of the development of the drapers' gild in London concluded that such vacant properties were colonised from the early 1350s by new businessmen taking advantage of the weakening monopoly by London merchants and purchasing the larger properties beyond the traditional gild core.[470] In other larger towns it is clear that some level of contraction could be blamed on plague. Of up to 280 dwellings in the city of Gloucester rented from Llanthony priory, it is quite clear that sixty (22 per cent) had become vacant in the years after the initial outbreaks of the plague. Half of these were the poorer cottages in the suburb beyond the South Gate, from which it is speculated that survivors of the plague moved to available and better located intramural properties.[471]

In Norwich, of ninety-one shops, stalls and tenements listed in a 1346 rental, forty-six had changed hands before 1357 and twenty-seven (29 per cent) were still vacant in that year.[472] In Coventry, it has been noted that the increase in property deeds (from fifty-seven surviving in the Coventry archives for 1348 to 177 in 1349) was accompanied by an increase in the use of the term *quondam* (one-time) when referring to adjacent properties for locational purposes. Thus, rather than mentioning existing tenants, the deeds referred to those who formerly held the properties. This usage went up from 21 per cent in 1348 to 46 per cent in 1349, hinting at a significant increase in the prevalence of empty properties. In Oxford, many halls formerly used for student accommodation lay empty immediately following the first outbreak, a picture supported by evidence of decaying buildings and vacant plots.[473] In many other towns, the decrease in rents gathered by religious institutions hints at the same story. Henry Knighton's chronicle noted that 'after the plague many buildings both large and small, in all the cities, boroughs and townships, decayed and were utterly razed to the ground'.[474] This glut of urban property may have impacted on the size of the properties in London. St Martin's seld, a covered market in the parish of St Pancras Soper Lane, contained twenty-one plots in 1250; by 1360 it comprised eleven larger plots, some of which were now shops with rooms above.[475]

However, this picture of contraction is complicated by the fact that an interest in speculative building activities remained and indeed increased in certain areas of the city and surroundings. The wealthy merchants Adam Fraunceys and John Pyel had, in August 1348 (thus just before the plague), contracted with the prioress of St Helen's Bishopsgate to demolish certain houses between the high road on the west and the convent garden and cemetery on the east; the aim was to build a new house and a block of five two-storey shops along the street. Despite the fact that the programme of building works ran throughout the months of the epidemic, the scheme had by December 1349 expanded to create eight shops and two houses. Before 1373, Fraunceys also built a block of at least six shops immediately east of the Austin friary in Broad Street. Other city projects included considerable redevelopment by the dean and chapter of the area south of St Paul's Cathedral on the sites of the cathedral brewery and bakery, in 1369–70, comprising one range of twenty shops with cellars and another of eighteen shops with cellars; and a block of five shops and houses built on Addle Lane in 1383 by Thomas Carlton, a borderer.

In Southwark in the 1370s there was clear evidence of similar large-scale building along Bermondsey Street and Tooley Street. In the latter, in 1373, a master carpenter was contracted by the prior of Lewes to build eleven jettied shops adjacent to the gatehouse of the prior's house in explicit imitation of the row built by Adam Fraunceys. At Westminster, rows of shops appeared in the precinct from 1354, and the site of the almonry was redeveloped by the almoner in successive blocks between 1357 and 1387, resulting in some thirty-four shops along the south side of Tothill Street. Subsidence required one shop to be raised on a new clay platform, indicating the relative simplicity of the buildings. These unitary, purpose-built developments were clearly not the only kinds of construction going on in the metropolis, but their appearance suggests a demand for a new kind of commercial property. There appears to be no evidence for new projects of this particular kind beyond 1400 for about a century, suggesting that it was a phenomenon associated with certain conditions and opportunities.[476]

Archaeological evidence for change to the city's topography is not at all clear: truncation of the majority of floor levels by more recent building activities generally leaves just foundations, rubbish pits and cesspits, making it rather hard to develop any coherent picture of the changes in the late fourteenth-century building pattern. Closer analysis of cesspit disuse alongside documentary evidence for the plots may well reveal more of a pattern of change or indeed continuity. In summary, it may be possible to envisage a contrasting picture of a far less crowded city and one with many new faces, displaying some decay and vacancy alongside bold, new and sometimes extensive redevelopment.

The plague might also have had an effect on the administration and governance of the city. Wider impacts on royal government included a reduction in experienced administrative staff through significant losses of the most senior officials in Chancery (three out of twelve clerks of the 1st grade died in both the first and second outbreaks), the Exchequer and the royal household. Longer-term changes in property rights, the Crown's approach to taxation, legislative controls over employment and appointments in county administration may all have been encouraged or hastened by the effects of the epidemics, even if some of the national labour market controls may have been adopted and adapted from pre-plague attempts by the city authorities at market regulation and enforcement.[477] However, these changes affected the whole nation, not specifically London. The demographic pressure induced by successive waves of plague certainly did have an impact on the stock from which the ruling city elite were drawn, and the basis for one of the city's more important codifications of its customs and regulations, the *Liber Albus* (dated 1419), makes this issue plain:

> when, as not unfrequently happens, all the aged, most experienced, and most discreet rulers of the royal City of London have been carried off at the same instant, as it were, by pestilence, younger persons who have succeeded them in the government of the City, have on various occasions been often at a loss from the very want of such written information, the result of which has repeatedly been dispute and perplexity among them as to the decisions which they should give.[478]

This change in the status quo was also evident in the evolution of burial customs of the aldermen, and was in the same volume placed firmly at the door of the plague:

> For it is matter of experience that even since ... 1350, at the sepulture of Aldermen the ancient custom of interment with baronial honours was observed ... But by reason of the sudden and frequent changes of the Aldermen and the repeated occurence of pestilence, this ceremonial in London gradually died out and disappeared.[479]

These observations, compiled by Richard Whittington, Mayor of London, provide a powerful sense of the impact of a high mortality rate on the preservation of experience and learning among the ruling class of the city, and suggest that an old order had passed with the plague. The elite were primarily drawn from the merchant class and merchant families now rarely survived for more than three generations in the male line.[480]

Competition for apprentices for the gilds which these merchant families ran became fiercer as a result of the plague. The devastating mortality rate experienced among apprentices in companies such as the Goldsmiths' (see Chapter 3) appears to have seriously exacerbated a problem of depressed numbers in the early 1340s. Analysis of a sample of gild ordinances shows that prohibition of 'enticement' or poaching of apprentices was specified in 56 per cent of cases (14/25) between 1344 and 1400, relaxing to just 14 per cent (4/28) in the period 1451–1500.[481] Competition, already significant when the plague struck, grew much fiercer in its wake and required regulation and management. As well as prohibitive measures, customary entry charges fell as gilds moved to encourage a greater uptake of positions. The grocers' fee for taking on apprentices was 20s in 1345, a sum which had plummeted to 3s 4d by 1376.[482] Younger starting ages (between 10 and 14) seem to have been permitted in the second half of the fourteenth century, and greater opportunities for the apprentices may be responsible for the fifty cases of absenteeism recorded in the surviving Mayor's Letters between 1350 and 1370.[483] Such cases also indicate that civic authorities were investing considerable time after the plague helping masters to recover apprentices who had left before completing their contracts, in contrast to the position beforehand.[484]

Overall, the strategies employed to maintain numbers seem to have worked – despite dips, the average enrolment of the Goldsmiths' Company was nineteen between 1334 and 1400, and seventeen between 1400 and 1500. Those who survived appear to have been able to reap the rewards: nearly 75 per cent of apprentices enrolled in the Goldsmiths' Company had taken on their own apprentice within eight to sixteen years of enrolment, compared with under half in the last quarter of the fourteenth century.[485]

There is some evidence for rapid change in certain craft trades which is suggestive of a link to the Black Death. London's trade in monumental brasses went through a process of rationalisation from a number of smaller entities to two big workshops which emerged in the second half of the 1350s, and for the next half-century these two firms would command a very large share of the English market overall. The first decade of this transformation may have been affected by skills loss, since minor compositions and not major monuments formed the principal output until around 1360.[486] Pottery trading in the London area also appears to have undergone a significant change, with pottery industries formerly used commonly in the capital all but vanishing from the scene and being replaced by new products.[487] Such transformations in industries would be unsurprising results of the high mortality of trained and experienced craftsmen, and it is probable that changes can be identified through closer examination of other London crafts and industries.

Civic ordinances and customs can provide a useful snapshot of changing habits and behaviours. Trading standards and controls were already in place in the city long before the advent of the plague, but there certainly seems to have been a transformation in the regulation of the city dress code, which was not governed by wider royal decree. In January 1352 the mayor and aldermen noted that 'common lewd' women had 'of late' begun to dress themselves in the manner 'of good and noble dames and damsels of the realm', and issued an order that neither resident nor visitor of lesser standing should wear any garments trimmed with fur, lined with sandal, buckram or samite, by day or night, in winter or summer, 'so that all folks, native or strangers, may have knowledge of what rank they are'. Forfeiture of the offending garment and/or prison were the punishments for transgressors.[488]

Of itself, there seems to be no direct link to pestilence since negative observations about the change in fashion appear prior to 1348, along with dire warnings about the misfortune that would befall such sins of pride; but what is important is that two subsequent chroniclers of the 1360s saw the wearing of indecent clothing as a specific cause for the wrath of God in the form of pestilence, and one Westminster monk, John of Reading, appears to echo Whittington's sentiments of a lost world order when he emotionally connected these outlandish fashions with a collapse of moral virtue and the readiness with which men and women would now consort with strangers, deflower virgins, and 'pervert every convention, decency and standard'.[489] Sumptuary laws of 1363 enacted into legislation similar controls to those city regulations of 1351, establishing ownership in London (and other towns) of £1,000 or more in goods and chattels to be the equivalent of esquires and gentlemen with £200 worth of land in terms of the dress code.

Women in London were subject to other kinds of control in the later fourteenth century. The pillory, a high wooden platform in Cheapside reached by a ladder upon which stood a frame that constrained the body in an extremely uncomfortable manner, was known to be in use from at least 1310, but the Letter Books and other sources mention only eight examples of its use between that date and the outbreak of plague in 1348. In contrast, no less than seventy-three cases are registered between 1350 and 1400 (59 per cent of all 125 cases identified between 1310 and 1500). Either crime was rife or the detection of cases and their prosecution was much more rigorous. Of these seventy-three cases, sixty-three were men, committed for one or more hours for a range of crimes including deception, impersonation of officials, cheating, theft, selling counterfeit or putrid goods, oath-breaking and prostitution. However, ten cases (13.6 per cent) were women, punished for a similar range of crimes, and of these, nine were sent to a specific type of pillory or punishment structure called the thewe, about which we know very little.

The thewe seems to have been a pillory specifically built for women, or perhaps a form of ducking stool. It is first mentioned in 1364 when Alice de Caustone, an ale-seller, had been caught thickening the bottom of a quart measure with pitch covered with rosemary to defraud buyers.[490] The pillory (and presumably thewe) were not simply irritating, stressful and humiliating punishments. A case in 1350 brought against seventeen men and five women for forestalling poultry (selling it before it arrived at the regulated market) made clear that one, previously convicted, would be pilloried while the remaining twenty-one would be let off with prison as it was their first offence. It is clear that the pillory was considered worse than a prison sentence. A specific focus on the punishment of women is also hinted at by the bequest by Thomas Gauder of money to both a house of women and a house of felons at Newgate.[491] There is, therefore, a sense that regulation and punishment had become much more of a public focus and that within this new regime, the transgressions of women had been specifically singled out. The influx of many new families as a result of the plague losses, and the perceived transformation of the old order in consequence, may have stimulated this need to establish control.

This attempt to exert controls extended to those who may not have transgressed specific regulations, but who nevertheless appeared guilty of avoiding work and attempting to live by means of charity alone. As far as government was concerned, the need to maintain a cap on earnings and wages had to be met in part by the increase in labour supply, at a time when this was in very short supply. The Ordinance of Labourers, enshrined in statute in 1351, encouraged disapproval of the 'sturdy beggars' – the undeserving poor – and subsequent city regulations made it an offence for those who could work to avoid it. Furthermore, those tempted to help them should be dissuaded, even forcefully through penalties of their own.[492] The reduction in dole money for major obituaries at Westminster has already been suggested as a result of this change in attitude (see Chapter 3), and this shift in emphasis may have triggered a change in the way hospitality, almsgiving and care for the sick manifested itself physically, through the arrangement and architecture of almonries and infirmaries.

The almonry of Westminster Abbey provides an important example of this. From 1290, the almonry was marked as a space separate from the abbey by a ditch and hedge. Principal buildings were visible from Tothill Street to the north and access was relatively uncontrolled. After 1350, the range of shops and houses described earlier, and, significantly, a gatehouse, came to line the street frontages and the space became highly controlled and inward-focused. It has been argued that this was as a result of the monks responding to the new ideology where the focus was shifting (a) to the concept of a deserving poor (and thus by implication exclusion of the undeserving poor), and (b) towards greater emphasis on resident beneficiaries.[493]

The move towards residential charity is mirrored by a shift in the monastic infirmaries from day care to in-patient care previously described at abbeys such as Westminster,[494] another change which can reasonably be ascribed to the effects of the plague. Subdivision of monastic dormitory halls into small, private rooms is well recounted and the process had begun well before 1348, but the plague may well have had a direct hand in similar evolution of the infirmary hall (and indeed the hospital hall). This has been dated generally to the period after 1350,[495] supported by archaeological evidence from sites in the London region. At the Augustinian priory of Merton in Surrey, about 6 miles south-west of the city, a very deliberate subdivision of the infirmary hall into partitioned rooms with tiled floors measuring 3.7m by 2.4m has been dated to the 1360s or 1370s, as has the insertion of timber screens at Waltham Abbey, Essex. At Westminster, documentary and architectural evidence indicates that the new infirmary, begun around 1360 and completed before 1390, provided chambers for all the beds.[496]

Examination of the care of Westminster monks in the infirmary between 1297–1355 and 1381–1417 may shed light on the timing for this change. Infirmarers' records show that the custom of providing a pittance to monks visiting the infirmary ceased for day-patients some time between 1354 and 1380. Thereafter, only in-patients received this sum of money: the concept of day-patients appears to have vanished. The time that in-patients spent there changed considerably from that seen before the plague, and indeed from that witnessed in the immediate aftermath. The median duration of in-patients' spells in the infirmary was twenty-two days in the first half of the fourteenth century, but had dropped to nine days in the second half; while 50 per cent of the spells in the earlier period had lasted between fourteen and sixty-three days, for the later period this had significantly reduced to between six and fourteen days. Treatment was therefore intensified at once by focusing much more on in-patient care, and yet significantly reduced in that those who did require such care were no longer permitted to stay there as long as they once had. Pressure on a vastly reduced convent to keep the abbey going may have been a key factor.[497] Such a move away from day care towards more intensive in-patient care may have catalysed redevelopment of the infirmary here and at other monastic houses in London to include separate chambers.

Monasteries and hospitals were not the only sources of charity. Individual gifts and bequests were hugely important in this regard. It is possible to examine the trends in pious and charitable bequests from the Husting wills and to consider the degree to which the concept of the deserving poor was reflected in the gifts left by well-meaning Londoners. Care must be given to the changing character of the wills themselves in the 1340s, but it is clear from a key study of testamentary behaviour that Londoners gave consistently more to the poor as the century progressed, and a high point of giving was in the decade after the first outbreak. This giving often took place at the graveside of the benefactor on the day of their funeral. Each pauper attending the funeral might get ½d or 1d, but the overall sums could be quite significant: for example, woolmonger Thomas Broun (d. 1357) and Richard de Walsted (d. 1366) both left 20 marks to be distributed in 1d lots, thus allowing for up to 3,200 poor people to benefit.

This form of charity was intended even by those caught up in the plague. In 1361 clerk Walter de Kent left 20s to be split in ½d portions suggesting he hoped 480 paupers would benefit; Hugh Peyntour's will drawn up in the same year similarly left ½d to 1,000 poor men. But former mayor, Richard de Kislingbury, eclipsed even these gifts by leaving £60 to be divided among the poor – at 1d each this would have benefited 14,400 paupers – and 9½ sacks (3,458lb in weight) of wool to be divided as one fleece per pauper. As a fleece may weigh as much as 12lb, this might have provided for 288 paupers.[498] We know that this kind of distribution did occur en masse as the wills suggest, since the Coroners' Rolls recorded the crushing to death in 1332 of fifty-two paupers as a result of crowding at the gate to Blackfriars during the distribution of money from Henry Fingrie's will.[499]

Some bequests were more particular, donating money to poor women, poor girls for marriage portions, or to poor widows. This kind of charity was relatively infrequent, appearing in less than 1 per cent of wills before the *pestis secunda*. During and after 1361, this increases to nearly 2 per cent (see Fig. 15). This trend can be complemented by around 10 per cent frequency found in a sample of Prerogative Court of Canterbury wills for Londoners between 1400 and 1530.[500] Such a pattern may show that Londoners perceived a

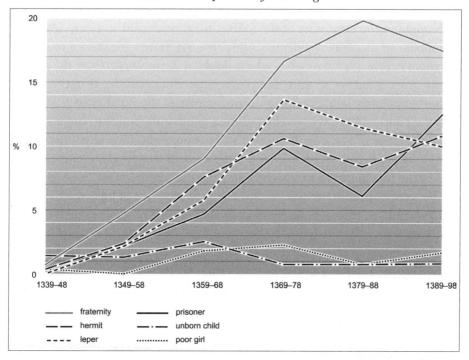

Fig. 15 Rates of change in particular bequests in the Husting wills to specific social and religious groupings. (Source: CHW, Vols 1 and 2)

diminishing in the marriage prospects of poor girls (nine cases), and, to a lesser extent, a stress on the ability of poor women, especially widows, to survive in the decades of major plague visitations (two cases). This sense of focus is strengthened when one considers that three of the wills were geographically specific. John Longe, a vintner, willed in 1361 money to support the marriage portions of poor girls throughout London; in the fourth outbreak, John Herlawe's will of October 1375 left money for the relief of the poor women and widows specifically living in Lime Street, rather suggesting that they were there in some numbers; and in 1390 William Trippelow left money to poor men and sick widows in five named city parishes. Such approaches are representative of an increasing focus on particular social groups or even individuals for charitable bequests in the second half of the century, a focus that is likely to represent a response to the plague.

Religious fraternities provided charity for members and their families should times prove hard, and also undertook wider charitable works within the community. Their role in providing some form of safety net for members' families and dependants in the first plague of 1348–9 has already been discussed, but the popularity of such groups increased significantly throughout the remainder of the fourteenth century, and, it seems clear, in response to successive epidemics. Only five fraternities are known to have existed before 1348, a number which doubled during 1349. Over the next fifty years, a further seventy-four fraternities were established in the city, their popularity witnessed by a major increase in the number of testators at the court of Husting who bequeathed goods and money to them.[501] As a percentage of the overall number of Husting wills, individuals making such bequests rose steadily from 4.8 per cent in the decade immediately after the first outbreak to a high of 19.8 per cent in the 1380s (see Fig. 15). The most popular fraternities to leave bequests to were St John the Baptist, for the gild of tailors, in St Paul's Cathedral (a total of 12.5 per cent of all 128 separate bequests recorded between 1338 and 1398), the fraternity of Salve Regina in the church of St Magnus the Martyr (7 per cent), and the drapers' fraternity of the Blessed Virgin Mary in the St Mary-le-Bow (5.5 per cent).[502] While the rise of such fraternities, linked often to crafts and trades as well as to local parish churches, was not solely precipitated by the successive waves of plague, it has been noted that it was 'not by chance that every set of fourteenth-century London fraternity ordinances specifies in great detail the burial obligations of its members, and that the Black Death at least provided incentive, and means for formation of parish fraternities';[503] gifts to such bodies ensured that the charity was focused quite particularly on the testators' neighbours, craft colleagues or friends.

Charitable bequests to assist poor hermits, anchorites and anchoresses also rapidly increased during the plague decades. These lone religious men and women, usually attached to churches, were reliant entirely on the generosity of the community. Hermits were able to leave their cells and undertake good works on behalf of the community, while anchorites and anchoresses were effectively confined, spending their lives in prayer. They were neither numerous nor widespread in London but they must have been well known. Husting wills before 1341 would not normally make any reference to them, since testators generally supported them with pecuniary bequests which were not included in the will until after this date. The great majority of the wills did not specify individual recluses, preferring presumably to leave the choice of beneficiary to the executor. These normally thus stated that a sum of money was to go to each anchorite and hermit of London, for example.

Some were much more specific, however, and from these we learn that there were anchorites associated with the churches of St Benet Fink and St Peter Cornhill (by 1345), St Giles Cripplegate (1348), St Lawrence Jewry, St Botolph Bishopsgate and Charing Cross (by 1361), the Swan's Nest (east of the Tower of London, by 1371), St Giles leper hospital (1373), and St Katherine's hospital by the Tower (a friar, John Ingram, by 1380). A hermit was resident at the chapel at the Newchurchehawe cemetery at West Smithfield by 1361.[504] Anchoresses and 'female recluses' are also mentioned.

Altogether, seventy-six bequests were made between 1345 and 1398, so charity was relatively rare; but, as with the fraternities, the frequency rises from less than 2 per cent of wills in the decade 1349–58, to a steady average of 10 per cent in the last three decades of the century. The reputation of lone religious recluses lay in their particular intercessory powers – their prayers were seen to be potent, even among other forms of religious intercession – and here, surely, lies the reason for their increasing popularity in the wake of the visible sign of heavenly displeasure that was the pestilence.

Another group increasingly, and perhaps surprisingly, favoured with personal charitable bequests was London's lepers. Fear of infection from the disease did, of course, exist prior to the pestilence. As early as 1277, the city forbade any lepers within the walls, and Edward III's edict of 1346 requesting the removal of lepers from the city and suburbs made it clear that royal concern was in combating 'the evils and perils which from the cause aforesaid may unto the said city, and the whole of our realm'. The impact of this edict is unknown, but following the first outbreak, the city felt able to use the concerns about mixing lepers with healthy citizens to attempt to argue for the replacement at St Giles leper hospital of (apparently healthy) members of the Order of St Lazarus with leprous Londoners in 1354; evidence of other attempts to restrict the entry of lepers followed in the 1370s. In 1372 a leprous baker was expelled from the city after being 'oftentimes before … commanded by the Mayor and Aldermen to depart from the City'; on 27 August 1375 (so at the end of the fourth outbreak) a further city edict saw gate porters charged with ensuring no lepers entered the city, and managers at the Hackney leper hospital and the Lock in Southwark charged with not letting lepers leave those houses. In November 1375 the authorities proclaimed that 'no lazar shall go about in the said city … and that every constable and beadle shall have power to take such persons, and bring them to Cornhill and put them in the stocks'.[505]

The link between plague and the control of leprosy appears to have continued into the fifteenth century.[506] It could, therefore, be argued that the heightened awareness of the threat of contagion intensified efforts to segregate sufferers from the rest of society. It may be that there was a perceived link between episodes of plague visited upon a hapless populace by a wrathful God intent on punishment for sin, and the visible scourge of leprosy, itself considered to be a disease brought on by immorality and sin. However, the urgency with which the authorities appear to have prosecuted their control over access to the city by lepers needs to be examined against the broader backdrop of increasingly numerous bequests by citizens to improve the lot of these sufferers. An analysis of the calendar of Husting wills shows that specific bequests to lepers, or lazars as they were occasionally termed, only appear during the first plague outbreak of 1349. There are none earlier. During that outbreak, and the decade following, just under 2 per cent of all wills provided for lepers. This figure rose between 1359 and 1368 to 6 per cent, and then increased dramatically to 14 per cent by 1378. The numbers remained constant at about 10 per cent of Husting wills until *c.* 1400 (see Fig. 15). Thereafter, such bequests become very rare, but persist until the 1480s.

The importance of the three principal leper houses (the Lock just south of the Southwark urban settlement, the hospital of St Giles-in-the-Fields to the west of the city, and the leper hospital at Hackney, about 2 miles north of Bishopsgate), and the less-favoured hospital at St James Westminster, seems clear from such evidence, though it would need to be substantiated by a close analysis of the Archdeaconry and Commissary Court probates for the last two decades of the century. It is further supported from studies of Norwich, Yarmouth, Scarborough and Beverley which suggest an even greater and longer-lived popularity following the plague.[507] The increasing favour in which Londoners held lepers as objects of charity after the pestilence provides a balance to the regulatory controls under which sufferers were placed, and supports recent research suggesting that the common, essentially Victorian, vision of the terrifying, unclean, contagious bell-ringers is a too simplistic way of characterising medieval approaches to this tragic disease.[508] While a link between leprosy and pestilence may have been established, the inmates of the hospitals were the subject of pity and their intercessory prayers were considered to be highly effective.

The most tightly regulated and confined social group to benefit from changes in charitable giving after the first pestilence was that of prisoners. In common with others, we do not see major gift-giving at all before 1341 since the wills did not include pecuniary bequests, but a clear increase in charitable bequests can be seen over the plague period. London had five principal gaols by the late fourteenth century: Newgate, Ludgate, the Fleet (all dating to before the fourteenth century), and across the river in Southwark, King's Bench (from 1368) and Marshalsea (from 1373).[509] Conditions in London gaols were hard. Inmates were expected to live off their own means or charity, and if that was not forthcoming, it could spell disaster.

The Newgate ordinances of the early fifteenth century indicate that gaolers could and did intercept alms, and the (incomplete) Coroners' Rolls record fifty deaths within Newgate in the years 1322–6 and 1338–40, at least

two of which (in 1322) were from starvation. From the late fourteenth century, different zones existed in Newgate: imprisoned citizens had rooms with
privies and chimneys (men on the north side of the prison, women on the
south); foreigners and inferiors had 'less convenient cells' (in another part);
and those guilty of major crimes were incarcerated in the basement cells
(also on the south side).[510] Bequests to assist prisoners emerge for the first
time in the Husting wills in 1346, but rise sharply after the first outbreak, to
5 per cent in the 1360s – the decade of the second and third plagues – and an
average of about 10 per cent of all wills made between 1370 and 1400. This
form of charity became firmly established, appearing in an average of 25 per
cent of a sample of wills from the Prerogative Court of Canterbury covering
the period 1400–1530.[511]

The sums were sometimes significant. John de Pulteney, for example, left
4 marks annually to prisoners in Newgate. A link to the pestilence seems
to be confirmed by the fact that the rate of bequests for wills specifically
made within the months of the *pestis secunda* in 1361 was 11 per cent. The
motivation behind such charity seems to focus on the poverty of prisoners;
John Scorfeyn's personal concern in his will of 1389 was 'for poor prisoners,
more especially women, in Ludgate and Newgate'.[512] Citizens will no doubt
have been well aware of their perilous situation and several wills refer to the
redemption of poor prisoners, aiming to effect the release of those unable to
find the money to pay off their debts.

Developing in parallel with this shift in charitable bequests was an
increasing concern for the location and nature of burial. This manifested
itself at three levels: the first was in the selection of particular churches or
religious houses for burial; the second was in the decision to be buried
within the church or chapel, or outside; and the third was the degree of
precision provided for the burial. The clearest measure of change can be seen
in the number of people who specified a location at all. The Husting wills
only begin to mention burial location in 1275, but it is very rarely recorded
between then and about 1339 when the practice of stating a preference for a
particular church or religious house begins to gain popularity. From January
1347 through to the essential cessation of the first plague outbreak in July
1349, only 44 per cent of Husting will-makers specified where they wished
to be buried. Between August 1349 and March 1361, this figure rose dramatically to 74 per cent, rising again to 88 per cent during the second pestilence.
By the end of 1375 it had reached 96 per cent.

There seems little doubt that Londoners felt a greatly increased need to
express their choice of burial site. Of those naming their preferred church,
most felt the need to further specify either an intramural burial (averaging

67.7 per cent) or burial in a churchyard (27.4 per cent). This ratio seems not to have changed across the period in any meaningful way. Notable within this general trend is the rapid increase in popularity of St Paul's Cathedral, and especially the Pardon churchyard there. The name appears first in April 1349, but only one will (of 392 dated between 1 November 1348 and 1 August 1349) makes reference during the first plague; between the first and second plagues, the frequency rose to 2.5 per cent (4 of 160 wills between August 1349 and March 1361),[513] and during the three months of the second plague it jumped rapidly to 12.1 per cent (16 of 132 wills), remaining at over 9 per cent thereafter (to the end of the 1370s). This contrasts strongly with the frequency of such testators requesting burial in the new cemeteries founded at East and West Smithfield, where the numbers average less than 1 per cent throughout the fourteenth century, and suggests that the wealthy developed a preference for the city's mother church in times of crisis, rather than adopting the newer institutions founded to cater for those crises. The friaries were poorly represented: between 1348 and 1370 only eight testators chose them for burial. This is perhaps surprising, given the fact that 175 testators left bequests during the same period to the four principal friaries.[514]

An increasing number of testators specified burial adjacent to a family member or loved one. The frequency was just 10 per cent up to the end of the first outbreak, but doubled to 21 per cent in the following decade, and rose again during and after the second plague to 24 per cent. It reached a height of 30 per cent in the third plague, but then appears to have fallen away to 12 per cent until the end of 1377. A comparative study on a sample of the Commissary Court wills from 1380 to 1541 concluded that between 18 and 60 per cent of testators identified a specific burial location;[515] so it may be that burial preference became more frequently expressed in other documents than the Husting enrolments.

The instructions could be very specific, requesting burial within the same tomb as a relative. In the case of John de Rothyng, a vintner, this was taken to considerable extremes. In his will dated 23 May 1375 he requested burial in St James Garlickhythe in the centre of the belfry floor and desired that the bodies of his mother and father be removed from their current location and buried with him.[516] Possibly the fragmentation of families as a result of the disaster elicited a strong response for survivors to ensure that they were reunited in death, if not necessarily during life. Noble dynastic mausolea were already well known in major churches across the land, but it might be argued that the plague provided a significant impetus for the development of family plots and vaults for the post-epidemic merchant and artisan classes.

Preparation for the afterlife, for some, involved the foundation of chantries where Masses for the souls of the founder and their family might be sung on a regular basis. Some had elaborate chapels built to house them, within or connected to a church; others were conducted at specified altars within the church. Some were perpetual, involving the allocation of property to generate income to pay for chaplains; others were funded by fraternities from year to year, and more were temporary, paid for by a bequest of money to purchase Masses for a specified period, often one year. The impact of the Black Death was ultimately complex. The national picture of perpetual chantries is one where the plague acted to greatly decrease the number of foundations. Studies of alienation in mortmain (the requirement for a royal licence to pass property to the Church) have shown that there was a dramatic reduction in the foundation of perpetual chantries in England following 1348. This national picture appears to be confirmed by specific studies of chantries in St Paul's Cathedral. Of eighty-four chantries founded in the cathedral between 1200 and 1548, sixty predate the plague; only seven were founded in the first fifty years after 1349. Noteworthy are the three chantries founded during 1349 as a direct result of the plague, but the trend is clear. Here, though, the plague must be seen as a contributor not the cause, for pressure was already apparent on the space available for new chantries and concerns about the impact of chantries on parish livings.

The plague brought a shortage of priests and in 1370 six chantries were vacant at St Paul's, a situation resolved only by a major amalgamation of chantries in 1391. The impact was therefore two-fold: a drop in foundation rate and a reduction in the number of existing chantries.[517] This is not, however, to say that chantry foundation as a whole decreased. A study of the bequests to chantries in the Husting wills shows that from 1259 to 1348, a total of 450 wills made mention of chantries (perpetual and temporary), an average of five wills per year. From 1349 to 1370, 383 wills made mention of chantries – an average of seventeen per year. This increase is partly skewed by the inclusion from 1341 of pecuniary bequests in Husting wills, but the trend is undoubtedly genuine.

More people left money to a greater number of temporary chantries, rather than providing larger grants to single long-term institutions. A related phenomenon appears after 1349 of large numbers of Masses being requested. To the 10,000 Masses of William de Thorneye (see Chapter 2) can be added the example of Johanna Cros, who left bequests to both plague chapels, to 'chantries' for the souls of her and her family, and for 11,000 Ave Marias and 11,000 paternosters to be said. In effect, the temporal dimension of a chantry foundation was being eschewed in favour of the quantity of intercession.[518]

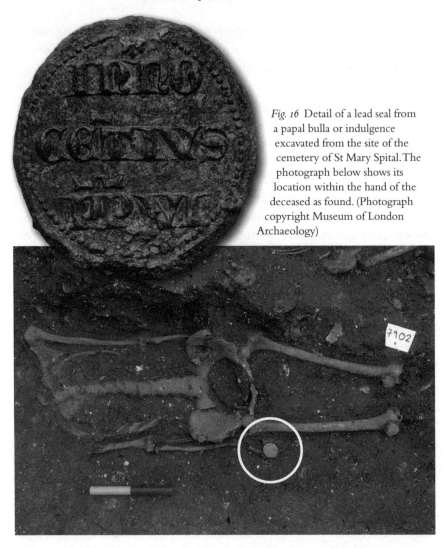

Fig. 16 Detail of a lead seal from a papal bulla or indulgence excavated from the site of the cemetery of St Mary Spital. The photograph below shows its location within the hand of the deceased as found. (Photograph copyright Museum of London Archaeology)

Overall, therefore, the pattern of chantry support shifted significantly in response to the plague, tending away from perpetual foundations towards more immediate and more intense approaches to intercession and com-memoration: faith in long-term stability appears to have been weakened.

Burial practice itself may have changed in the wake of the 1348 outbreak, probably reflecting another stratagem for ensuring intercession for the soul. The use of papal bullae as amulets or charms to accompany the dead has been described elsewhere (see Fig. 16),[519] but the importance of the rite here is that the majority of known examples date to the period 1350–70. The link between the discovery of these lead seals in graves, the rise of Chaucer's despised pardoners in the later fourteenth century, and good evidence in the same period for the counterfeiting and import of such seals, suggests a lively market in the purchase of talismans to reduce the pain of Purgatory or to ward off sudden death.

These observations on the social impacts of the plague are only part of the story. The impact on London's economy and its relationship with its markets and its hinterland, and the longer-term changes wrought in demographic structure and population movement, have not been the subject of this study, but the potential must surely be there. The examples of social change suggest that it is reasonable to assert that the plague triggered a fundamental shift in charity and good works, linked to strategies for securing the salvation of the soul, but also, clearly, linked to simple empathy and sympathy for those less fortunate than the benefactors themselves. It is dangerous to generalise, but there is a sense that while better-off Londoners were perhaps more choosy about what they gave and to whom, they gave more than they had before the plagues, and they placed an increasing value on family, friends and neighbours through their ties with the parish, the fraternities, and through their choices for the hereafter. And this pattern developed in the face of disasters which saw whole families extinguished and neighbourhoods transformed. If there is a single word which captures the character of the city through this extraordinary trial, it is resilience.

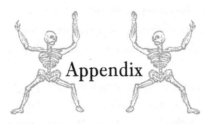

Appendix

LONDON'S CONTRIBUTION TO UNDERSTANDING THE BLACK DEATH

The Nature of the Pestilence: Current Debates

THIS BOOK does not set out to prove whether the great mortality or pestilence, as it was known to those who suffered it, was bubonic plague, anthrax, typhus, haemorrhagic fever or some other disease. However, the London evidence can contribute to the debate in this contested arena, since it would appear to point away from the argument for bubonic plague and towards something else. It is impossible for this author in this volume to attempt a full critical survey of all published theories on the Black Death and its character, but in order to provide the basis for any such argument, a summary of the different approaches and theories is necessary; it is hoped that the key elements of the various arguments have been acceptably precised here.[520]

The pestilence was, for the vast majority of schoolchildren and researchers alike, bubonic plague. This has been the accepted identification of the Black Death for most of the twentieth century, since the outbreak of a plague in Hong Kong in 1894 by a team including Alexandre Yersin: the bacterium was eventually called *Yersinia pestis* after him. In the early 1900s, the link between the bacillus, fleas and rats was made, and in 1914 the mechanism which caused rat fleas to attack humans.[521] Yersin himself made the first connection between the nineteenth- and early twentieth-century outbreak of bubonic plague and the medieval scourge, linking it also to the even earlier outbreak in *c.* AD 540 known as the Justinian plague.[522]

The main arguments in favour of this being the medieval pestilence are based around its observed characteristics – the common presence of bubos in most of the chronicles and many medical observations, and the similarities of other symptoms and of the progress of the disease. Variants in description (such as the spitting of blood, or of victims dying within hours almost unmarked) are explained through the presence of three varieties of plague caused by *Yersinia*: bubonic, where the infection passes from the bite site into the lymphatic system causing bubos; pneumonic, where the bacteria are transported from the bite site to the lungs causing secondary pneumonia; and septicaemic, where the infection is directly into a vein effectively allowing rampant bacterial reproduction and assault before the body can mount any effective defence. Interpersonal infection risk in all cases is low. The disease can be moved effectively around urban and rural areas by the presence of rats and the capacity for people to transport infected fleas in grain or clothing.[523] Death rates for nineteenth and twentieth-century outbreaks can be as high as 35 per cent in particular localised settlements, but at a regional level seldom exceed 3 per cent.[524]

The requirements for a bubonic plague outbreak are a suitable rodent vector (the black rat is the usual suspect) and a flea population that is active (most of the year except winter).[525] A forceful supporter of the bubonic plague argument is Professor Ole Benedictow, who has attempted a detailed reconstruction of the spread of the first plague outbreak across Europe in terms of a sequence of epizootics (where first the rat population in a given area contracts and perishes from the disease, and then, as the infected fleas seek new food, creates epidemics within the associated human population), spread and established by human transport of rat and flea vectors. His assertion that modern bubonic plague and experiences of its outbreaks are directly comparable with those of medieval pestilence has, however, been questioned, and his particular use of chronicle sources to support an epidemiological analysis of spread is considered by some to be rather too risky.[526]

Support for the bubonic model has been offered on the basis of the reported extraction of ancient *Yersinia* DNA (aDNA) from the dental pulp of skeletons recovered from cemeteries argued to be from plague outbreaks, with the interpretation that this evidence concludes the debate. However, questions have been raised about the basic assumptions underlying the samples used for the aDNA research, and some scientists have questioned the possibility of contamination of some samples. A test to obtain aDNA from skeletons from the London East Smithfield plague cemetery (among others) proved negative, although many other kinds of aDNA were recovered; but a more recent study of the mid-fourteenth-century mass burials excavated at Hereford Cathedral (and other European sites) has again identified the bacillus.

Correspondence among researchers demonstrates the difficulties in using such approaches to obtain a definitive answer.[527] There are two principal issues with claims, for example by Haensch et al., that aDNA discovery 'ends the debate about the etiology of the Black Death'. The first is the assumption during sample selection for testing that mass burial equates to plague ('mass' has been as few as two burials in a single grave in one study). This is unsupportable, since outbreaks of infectious disease other than plague must have been extremely common in the medieval period, and we know that severe famine caused mass deaths on at least two occasions (in the mid-thirteenth century and in the early fourteenth century). The second is that the discovery of *Y. pestis* aDNA simply tells us that the plague bacillus was present; to offer categorical assertion that it was the agent of the 1348 disaster requires us to prove both its prevalence in skeletal material firmly tied to the outbreak, and in addition its absence in skeletons dating before this date. One thing that all researchers seem to agree on is the need for suitable independent and blind testing in order to solve the issue.

The fit of modern bubonic plague to the documented evidence for the pestilence has always been problematic to a degree. As early as 1893 (and thus a year before Yersin started his work in Hong Kong), Gasquet noted of the 1348 outbreak that 'together ... with the usual characteristics of the common [meaning bubonic] plague, there were certain peculiar and very marked symptoms, which although not universal, are recorded very generally in European countries'. These were, he said, 'gangrenous inflammation of the throat and lungs, violent pains in the region of the chest, the vomiting and spitting of blood, and the pestilential odour coming from the bodies and breath of the sick'. He concurred with Charles Anglada, a Parisian physician, who in his study of extinct and new diseases published in 1869 expressed a 'profound conviction that the Black Death stands apart from all those which preceded or followed it'.[528] This recognition of the highly unusual nature of the 1348 pestilence was set aside as the post-Yersin bubonic model became firmly established. Nonetheless, subsequent researchers into the impact and effects of the pestilence, while content to accept bubonic plague as the culprit, continued to have some problems with making the evidence fit the diagnosis. In 1963 historian J.M.W. Bean noted that the Black Death must have:

> contained a very considerable pneumonic element, a fact which is suggested by three of its features: first, the exceptionally high death rate; second, the descriptions by contemporary observers of the symptons which are nowadays met in pneumonic plague; and third, the fact that the Black Death raged in

winter as well as summer, so that many bubonic victims are likely to have contracted pneumonia and 'triggered off' pneumonic outbreaks.[529]

The inherent problem with this analysis was recognised just a few years later, in 1970, by the bacteriologist J.F.D. Shrewsbury, who noted that 'the pneumonic plague cannot occur in the absence of the bubonic form and it cannot persist as an independent form of plague'. He went further:

> Our modern knowledge of the bionomics [of the rat flea] explains why in medieval England epidemics usually erupted towards the end of spring, rose rapidly to a peak of intensity in late summer or early autumn, collapsed or declined sharply with the arrival of autumn frosts, and were extinguished in or remained dormant throughout the winter months.[530]

Indeed, his whole thesis comprised a sustained attack on the documentary evidence for high mortality and winter spread precisely because it did not fit the bionomics of rat and flea populations and the aetiology of bubonic plague. He argued for a range of coterminous diseases being responsible for the mortality seen in the fourteenth-century outbreaks.

Despite the inherent contradictions that this kind of situation gives rise to, it was to be another decade before a cautionary note was sounded. In 1979 Stephen Ell, undertaking an examination of more than 300 medieval plague accounts, concluded that the human flea, and thus human-to-human transmission, more closely fitted the bill.[531] Three years later, the risks associated with extrapolating modern plague experience backwards to the 1348–9 outbreak were raised by medical historian N.G. Siraisi,[532] and in 1984 the first co-ordinated confrontation of the bubonic model was mounted by zoologist Graham Twigg. In it he argued that the specific problems of the reproductive capacity of fleas in cold winters and cold climates, and the presence of appropriate rodents (i.e. the black rat) in appropriate numbers for them to prey on, were too great to be surmounted. He expressed doubts about whether the speed of transmission was consonant with the requirements of bubonic plague. The bubos and other symptoms described in the contemporary literature he thought were potentially associated with other diseases as readily as with bubonic plague. He also brought into play references to chroniclers who mentioned the death of larger animals as well as men, and concluded that the answer was more likely some form of disease of animals that also affected humans, and made a tentative case for anthrax, spread person-to-person.

Detractors from this view raised the issue of our ability to compare like with like, the dangers of using sources selectively, and the lack of any real evidence for widespread larger animal deaths in the plagues of the later sixteenth and seventeenth centuries. It was in one case also noted that the physicians of the day knew the difference between pestilence buboes and anthrax carbuncles.[533]

Bean rejoined the debate in 1982. Accepting bubonic plague as the agent, he reasserted that since there was undoubtedly a rapid spread of the disease during winter months, 'it was reasonable to assume ... there was pneumonic plague'. However, he recognised that if the plague had indeed assumed different seasonal characteristics (bubonic in summer, pneumonic in winter), we should expect to see different mortality rates – much higher in the areas affected in winter. The fact that this was not borne out in studies of summer mortality in Orvieto, Siena and San Gimignano (with mortality rates of 50 per cent or more) he sought to explain away by arguing that cities were at far greater risk.[534]

In 1986 the issue of the black rat itself came under scrutiny by David E. Davis, a zoologist at North Carolina State University. Following a survey of archaeological and documentary indications of rats and a consideration of the ecological requirements of *Rattus rattus*, he concluded that 'the accumulated evidence, interpreted by ecological and epidemiological methods, does not support the traditional view that black rats were responsible for the Black Death'. Subsequent studies concluded that the archaeological evidence for *Rattus* in the medieval period was more considerable than Davis had allowed for, but one French study raised the issue of the viability of the flea carrier itself:

> the rat population had gradually grown from a fairly restricted one in the early Middle Ages to a significant one in the 11th and 13th centuries. The rodents spread along the major highways explaining the very different geographical impact of the various plague epidemics of the early and late medieval periods. However, the mystery of the exact mechanisms by which plague spread has still not been entirely elucidated, since the Asian rat flea, *Xenopsylla cheopis*, whose role as vector was demonstrated by P.L. Simond [an early twentieth-century bubonic plague researcher], could not have survived in the temperate European climate.[535]

The role of rats came under increased pressure, this time from Iceland in 1996. This related to two plague outbreaks argued to be of the Black Death type, in 1402–3 and 1494–5, which may have resulted in more than 50 per cent mortality rates, and which were able to attack the human population even in winter. The researcher, Gunnar Karlsson, argues that there were no rats in Iceland at the time, and that in winter the plague spread rapidly into areas of the country which enjoy a mean temperature of 0°C at that time of year. He supported the view of an earlier scholar, Jon Steffensen, who had proposed that pneumonic plague, not bubonic plague, was the cause.[536]

A further alternative was proposed by Susan Scott and Christopher Duncan in 2001.[537] They had taken the very detailed documentary evidence from the outbreak of plague in Penrith, Cumbria, in 1597 and used analysis of this, in conjunction with wider epidemiological and environmental concerns over the identification of bubonic plague as the killer, to argue that whatever it was, the pestilence was transmitted person to person, had a long incubation period (around thirty-two days, allowing it to be spread widely before a plague event was obvious), and was haemorrhagic in nature. They adopted the term 'haemorrhagic plague'. They were also able to develop a simulated model of what should happen in terms of death rates and compare this with real late sixteenth- and seventeenth-century examples of plague outbreaks (assuming that these were the same as the Black Death itself, of course). The argument against bubonic plague as the culprit was based around the low speed of transmission of this disease, the impact of climate on rat and flea vectors, and the low mortality rate of modern bubonic plague in comparison with reported and inferred death rates during the medieval pestilence. As with Twigg, critics of this approach cited selective use of documentation.[538]

The most sustained published attack on the bubonic model, drawing on many of the specific concerns raised previously, has come from historian Sam Cohn.[539] His approach was essentially to deconstruct the century-old assumptions regarding the relationship between modern bubonic plague and the documentary evidence for the spread not only of the 1348–9 outbreak of pestilence, but the subsequent fourteenth-century outbreaks across Europe. In it he uses important new evidence for contemporary description and understanding of the plague from plague tractates, as well as assembling a formidable array of primary documentary evidence from wills and other quantifiable sources. He does not pretend to know what the disease was, but, like the pre-Yersin historians, he is certain that it was not the bubonic plague. His arguments against that diagnosis are well worth reading, but can be summarised as:

- The symptoms do not satisfactorily tie the disease down as bubonic plague.
- There is no contemporary report of elevated rat mortality (although there are chronicles reporting birds and sheep and other kinds of animals dying during the plague period).

– The mortality rates far exceed anything like modern bubonic plague.

– The seasonality of the outbreaks defy standard bubonic plague progression.

– The evidence for reducing mortality rates in successive outbreaks, combined with increasing proportions of child mortality, suggest increasing acquired immunity, something not possible for modern bubonic plague.

– In some well-documented Italian cities, epicentres of plague outbreaks were not associated with granaries as modern bubonic plague has been, but were associated with poor, artisan parishes.

– The pestilence struck regions where the rat/flea vectors could not have been present.

Also using documentary evidence, but bringing statistical analysis to bear on them, historical anthropologist James Woods, and colleagues from Pennsylvania State Universities and Georgetown University, re-examined the use of bishops' registers (recording the replacement dates of parish priests who had died) in the diocese of Coventry and Lichfield.[540] They discovered that the standard one-month estimate for the replacement used by most researchers actually varied considerably between a few days and several months, hiding the true dates of the plague's arrival at any given parish, and thus potentially underestimating the speed of transmission. They also found that hidden within the overall blanket of nine months (March to November 1349), in which the pestilence raged in the diocese, individual archdeaconries suffered in shorter bursts of four to six months, and noted that if this were true at archdeaconry level, the speed of transmission from parish to parish would almost certainly be faster again. This they saw as profoundly different from anything presented by the nineteenth/twentieth-century evidence, and as an argument against bubonic plague.

An unusual explanation for the plague has been presented by Mike Baillie, a palaeoecologist specialising in events dated in palaeoenvironmental sequences such as tree rings and ice-cores.[541] In 2006 he presented his idea that the Justinian and Black Death plague outbreaks were associated with very significant environmental and climatic changes, possibly as a result of comet strikes; what the plague was actually caused by he remains cautious about, but he believes it was air-borne (and not bubonic) and raises the possibility of biological pathogens being introduced into earth's atmosphere by the comets. Such a proposal, he recognises, will be seen as far-fetched by many, but the environmental markers he establishes for the fourteenth century are convincing and important for the study of this period.

One final twist to this swirl of debate and research has been the report that bubonic plague may actually be transmissible faster than previously thought. Researchers at the Division of Vector-Borne Infectious Diseases at the National Center for Infectious Diseases in Colorado conducted a study of an American carrier of bubonic plague (O. montana). In their words:

> in contrast to the classical blocked flea model, O. montana is immediately infectious, transmits efficiently for at least 4 days post-infection ... and may remain infectious for a long time because the fleas do not suffer block-induced mortality. These factors match the criteria required to drive plague epizootics as defined by recently published mathematical models.[542]

While this still requires a rodent or similar vector to produce the plague reservoir, the long incubation period and short infection window described in the existing bubonic model could be dismissed. If the disease was bubonic plague, the impact this research might have on, for example, Benedictow's carefully plotted chronology of spread and infection could be considerable. In any event, their acceptance that the characteristics of modern bubonic plague do not match at all well with the documentary evidence of past epidemics is important.

This short summary demonstrates the difficulties in getting a definitive identification. The capacity for pathogens to evolve, the variability of the primary documentary sources, and the complexities surrounding the science of the epidemiology and DNA character of the plague agent all present formidable challenges. However, further research into the evidence from specific cities, towns, villages and manors remains of the greatest importance in helping to solve this mystery.

A Consideration of the Evidence – The Plague's Arrival

The other great unknown about the plague, contingent of course on what caused it, is the definite timing of its arrival and the speed and manner of its spread across the country. Again, as a prelude to a consideration of London's contribution, it is necessary to look at current evidence. The most frequently deployed evidence comes from a range of medieval chroniclers. The advantage of this kind of source is that many had lived through, or were near contemporaries of, one or more of the outbreaks; some were eye-witnesses. The disadvantage is that there were differing concepts of truth within chronicles, used to impart separate messages to the reader,[543] and that the sources for such chronicles might rely on second- or third-hand information. The evidence is, therefore, not straightforward. Table 5 shows the range of dates in a selection of chronicles broadly contemporary with the time of the epidemic. Considerable variation exists bracketing a three-month period from late June to the end of September. There is also a disagreement over a south or west coast entry point. On this uncertain basis, scholars have ascribed different levels of dependability to the chronicles, from overall caution to confident assertion that a date in late June or early July must be accepted.[544] Most agree that the south coast, specifically Weymouth (Melcome), was the first port affected.

There are other more objective records which can be brought to bear. These fall into three categories. The first source is the evidence in the bishops' registers. These documents, kept by each bishop for his diocese, recorded among other matters the filling of clerical vacancies within the diocese, whether caused by resignation, cessation, exchange or death. The latter group, where they can be identified, are clearly of great significance in helping to track the plague, since abnormal clusters of vacancies may be taken to illustrate heightened mortality in a particular area. However, the dates recorded are of replacement of the rector or vicar, not of the death itself. To be able to use the evidence, we need to understand the lag between the two. This lag was the time it took to report a death to the episcopal authorities, identify a suitable replacement, institute him to the benefice and record the fact in the register. It has been generally estimated at between twenty-one and forty-two days, suggesting a standard period of thirty-five days to some.[545] However, closer examination of the register for the diocese of Coventry and Lichfield, unique in recording the actual dates of death for the clergy, shows that the median period was twenty-two days and that there are reasonable grounds for arguing that the earlier in the outbreak the death occurred, the shorter the lag.[546]

Dorset lay within the diocese of Salisbury and the bishop at the time was Robert Wyville (fl. 1330–75).[547] The earliest realistic contender for a plague-related institution was at West Chickerell (near Weymouth) on 30 September 1348. Prior to this, institutions were relatively infrequent and clustering was absent; afterwards, the frequency of institutions markedly increases in parishes and towns such as Warmwell, Dorchester and Wool from 9 to 24 October. If the vacancies were due to deaths, this would point (on the basis of the Coventry and Lichfield analysis) to deaths mounting from early September into October in the Weymouth/Poole area. Further institutions occurred in the Salisbury area (some 50 miles north-east) between 20 and 28 October.[548] There is good coherence in this distribution, providing the basis for estimating a general speed of spread of 1 mile to 1.5 miles per day.

Source	When Written	Suggested Plague Date	Outbreak Location	Reference
Geoffrey le Baker	1340s	Before 15 August 1348	A Dorset seaport	Thompson 1889a, 98–9
Ralph Higden	1341–52	24 June 1348	Bristol	Lumby 1882, 344–6
Robert of Avesbury	1340s and '50s	1 August 1348	Dorset	Thompson 1889b, 406–7
Eulogium (Malmesbury)	1350s	7 July 1348	Melcombe, Dorset	Haydon 1863, 213–4
John of Reading	1360s	After Midsummer 1348	*Not given*	Tait 1914, 106–10
Greyfriars of King's Lynn	1360s and '70s	21 June 1348	Melcombe, Dorset	Gransden 1957, 274
Thomas Stubbs	1373	30 September 1348	*Not given*	Raine 1886, 418
Anonimalle, St Mary York	1370s	1 August 1348	Bristol	Galbraith 1927, 30
Henry Knighton	1378–9	1348	Southampton	Martin 1995, 99

Table 5. Chroniclers' estimations of the date and location of the arrival of the plague in England.

Nevertheless, the uncertainty over the lag between vacancy and institution requires corroborative evidence. This exists to a degree in some surviving royal documents, particularly the Patent Rolls. Among many other items, these recorded the occasions of royal presentations of candidates for vacant churches in the king's hands. A church might enter royal control for one of two principal reasons at this time: the lord (secular or religious) may have died; or the religious house, having rights of presentation, may have been foreign (normally French), and thus its properties were sequestered by the Crown during the war. Either way, the king was entitled to propose his candidate for the vacancy, which the bishop either confirmed or not. The key point here is that the date of royal presentation lay somewhere after the vacancy/death but before the actual institution, so it acts to narrow down the date of death. Taking the Weymouth/Salisbury area of Dorset, we find a cluster of presentations between late September and mid-November 1348, none further than 20 miles from Weymouth: Dorchester on 20 September; Bincombe on 8 October; Bradford Peverell on the 16th; Piddlehinton on the 27th; Tolpuddle on the 30th; Portesham and Abbotsbury on 6 November; two churches in Wareham on the 8th and 12th, and on 13 November Owermoigne and Blandford.[549] These may well represent deaths from mid-September through to the beginning of November.

A further source of evidence is sometimes available from manorial documents. The estates of lords, bishops and monastic houses all required complex administrative and legal apparatus to account for production and to regulate the labour force working the land. Such apparatus gave rise to periodic documentation in the form of account rolls and court records. These survive in England better than in any other European country and, while their composition and survival are highly variable, they can provide exceptionally clear and objective information about the arrival and duration of the pestilence.

Where clerical vacancies occur in the same locale for which such manorial evidence exists, these documents can be used to 'anchor' the evidence from the registers. An example of how this type of evidence can assist comes from Gillingham in Dorset, 40 miles north of Weymouth. A recent discovery of a series of court rolls for three manors centred on Gillingham shows quite clearly that exceptional mortality was recorded during the first two weeks of October 1348.[550] Deaths peaked between 5 and 27 November (the dates of successive courts) but had effectively subsided by early February 1349. Two clerical vacancies in nearby Shaftesbury (just 4 miles south-east) were filled on 29 November and 10 December. Allowing for around twenty-two days' lag, these vacancies would have occurred between 7 and 18 November, agreeing remarkably well with the manorial documents. This timing appears consonant with further manorial evidence, this time from the manor of Curry Rivel, Somerset (also about 40 miles north-east of Weymouth), where numerous deaths were recorded in court rolls between 15 October and early December.[551]

Taken as a whole, there is a very strong impression that the plague made itself apparent in September at the earliest and developed rapidly through October and November. The implied later date for the plague's appearance makes much more understandable the letter of Ralph of Shrewsbury on 17 August (see Chapter 1), requiring preparation against an expected threat, and that of the Bishop of Winchester dated 24 October, establishing that the 'coastal' regions were, finally, under attack.

Other evidence previously offered in support of the chroniclers' summer date for the outbreak of plague can be readily refuted. Two detailed references have been published (and repeated) by way of proof and confirmation of the chroniclers that pestilence was abroad in July and August 1348 in Somerset and Dorset. The first stated: 'By the beginning of August [implying 1348], most of the tenants of Frome Braunch in Somerset were dead and there were other deaths in North and South Cadebury.' The reference, found in the Calendar of Inquisitions Post Mortem, is in fact to 1349.[552] The second recorded the 'statement that the king had noted in July 1348 that the mortality of men in the prebend of Bere Regis and Charminster in the present pestilence is so great that the lands thereof lie untilled'. This reference, found in the Calendar of the Fine Rolls, is again to July 1349.[553]

While more synthesis is clearly needed in this area, there is a strong possibility that the deadly character of the pestilence became apparent in September and not June or July 1348[554] and spread outward in October just as the season began to worsen and temperatures to drop. This implies that its speed of transmission into southern England was greater than has been previously entertained, and that this speed was not apparently unduly influenced by cooling temperatures.

The Experience of London & its Contribution to the Debate

Currently, the jury is still out on two key and linked debates: what the disease actually was, and the manner of its arrival and spread into England. London can contribute to these debates in a number of ways.

The first way in which the London study can inform this debate is over the issue of the rats themselves. Leaving aside for the moment the problem of Iceland, the bubonic model requires that the initial epizootic phase occurs for each rat colony before the fleas depart their dying hosts to begin the infection of humans. Archaeologists in London (and indeed across the UK) now routinely sample key stratigraphic groups (pit fills, ditch fills, cesspit fills, etc.) for environmental remains, using established sampling procedures which involve both the hand-collection and wet-sieving of bulk soil samples. Recovered through such procedures are the bones of fish, birds, amphibians and small mammals. Such tiny bones do not routinely survive, being readily susceptible to decay and destruction by natural processes, but the general incidence of rat bones (*Rattus rattus*) can be considered.

London has produced unequivocal evidence of the presence of *R. rattus* in the period both immediately before the outbreak of plague and during the later fourteenth century. Excavations adjacent to the medieval Guildhall have produced fifteen positively identified *R. rattus* bones from among a collection of discarded cat skeletons (used by furriers and skinners), scavengers no doubt, along with the remnants of red kites and crows. The yard deposits were dated to 1280–1350, and probably towards the latter date, since the yard also contains features associated with construction works on the Guildhall which were completed in the 1350s.[555] Four bones were located in a flood-prone area of New Palace Yard, Westminster, dated to *c.* 1230–1350.[556] In refuse dumps within the city ditch, eight *R. rattus* bones were recovered at

Aldersgate dated to 1350–1400; and four 'rat' bones (not specifically identi-fied as *R. rattus*) at Newgate dated 1340–1400.[557] Rat bones were recovered from a hearth in an undercroft of the substantial mansion house of Sir John de Pulteney (himself a victim of the 1349 pestilence), dated to the later four-teenth or early fifteenth centuries; and from fourteenth-century domestic rubbish dumps at the quay adjacent to Baynard's Castle. Two rat bones have also been recovered from the Augustinian priory of St Mary Merton, Surrey (about 7 miles south-west of the city), one from within the stone infirmary hall (dating to 1360–90) and one from the adjacent garden (1300–90).[558]

Further afield, a partial skeleton of a black rat was recovered from an ashy occupation layer around a hearth in the stone hall of a moated manor at Chalgrove, Oxon, dated to the late fourteenth or fifteenth centuries; rat bones were found at the Bishop of Winchester's manor in Witney, Oxfordshire, dating to the fourteenth century, and a similar partial skeleton was found in the guardroom of the inner ward of Barnard Castle in County Durham dated to 1330–1479. Finally, the presence of rats in a mid-fourteenth-century monastic setting is confirmed by references of payments made to rat-catchers at Durham Cathedral priory in 1347 and 1356.[559] One researcher claimed: 'There is nothing surprising about the almost complete exemption of the English nobility and landed class from "The Great Pestilence". It just hap-pened that the house-rat could not make itself at home in their castles.'[560] The evidence both from London itself and other sites across England refutes this.

There are, however, significant blanks in just the places we might expect to find the evidence – for example, many of the thirteenth- to fourteenth-century waterfront reclamation dumps which have been sampled but from which no rat bones have been identified. By definition, such deposits are normally waterlogged (encouraging excellent organic preservation), they are composed of dumped urban rubbish behind wooden or stone revet-ments (and so should be expected to contain disposal evidence of any mid-fourteenth-century mass rat deaths) and they are precisely the locations where many plague historians have posited that the impact would be the worst – along waterways. These references do not represent a comprehen-sive national survey but, as far as the bubonic model is concerned, it would appear that the black rat was present and reasonably widely distributed in and around the London region. But we cannot yet speculate on the size and number of colonies that may have existed, and thus the degree to which they could have supported a widespread epizootic. The evidence, patchy as it is, proves that rats were present, but not that they carried the plague.

The second contribution concerns the seasonality of the outbreak. We can be certain that deaths had not reached plague proportions in London by

25 October 1348 (when Edington wrote his letter in his Southwark palace, praying that his own city and diocese of Winchester be spared the impending onslaught from the coast). We can be equally certain that that scale had been achieved by 14 November (when the blanket indulgence to all London citizens was issued by the Pope). Depending upon its incubation rate, the infection probably established itself in the city no earlier than late September or early October. This is much later than the date provided, for example, by Benedictow (4 August), which he calculated from the earliest chronicled date of 29 September, including an eight-week period for the bubonic plague to become epizootic and then epidemic. This delay in development may be crucial in terms of the environmental argument.

If the plague was bubonic, and the biology of the black rat and the flea is as has been stated, we would have to accept that this winter was a particularly mild one, as below 10°C bubonic plague spread is significantly slowed. London's current average monthly temperature range does not exceed this figure from November through to March, and evidence from broader climate studies suggests that the fourteenth century saw deteriorating climatic conditions for much of northern Europe (and indeed globally), with oak growth rates at a consistently low level from the early 1340s for a decade, and one study of eastern England indicating at least three severe winters in the decade up to 1348.[561] So a mild winter does not appear to have been the case.

Fig. 6 (see p. 85), showing both the dates of writing and the dates of enrolment of wills, and the mortality rates for Stepney manor, establishes with as much certainty as can be hoped for that in the largest city in the land, the plague's transmission speed increased as London slipped into the grip of winter. The only previous attempt to integrate the progression of the pestilence through London with the environmental and seasonal requirements of the bubonic model proposed that the first epidemic manifestation emerged in later September, leading into a phase of infection among the poor, drawn out by the cool autumn months. This triggered a scare among the wealthy leading to a rise in will-making in November and December, and was followed by a full explosion of plague with the arrival of warm, spring weather.[562] The evidence from the Stepney manorial deaths refutes this 'considerable' time-lag between the onset of plague among the poor and the subsequent panic of the wealthy: the poor began to die exactly at the time when the richer began to draw up wills in exceptional numbers. The will enrolment trajectory matches very closely that of the will-making, and, taking the available evidence for lag between probate and enrolment, the likely death curve sits just three weeks later than the will-making curve. Therefore, the plague quite clearly escalated throughout the winter and had already peaked by Easter and the onset of warmer weather. This combination of circumstances does not appear to match the expected bubonic model. So for the traditional bubonic model to stand up we would have to accept that there were more rats than archaeological evidence is as yet offering, and that the winter was particularly mild. Even then, the chronology of the outbreak has been significantly revised.

This speed of transmission ought also to be considered in the light of the date at which the plague struck England as a whole (see above). Since official documentation suggests that the plague broke out in earnest possibly in late September and more certainly in October 1348, in a range of places from Dorset and north Devon right across to London, there would be insufficient time for the process of epizootic development in rat colonies, followed by spread into the human population, to allow for land-based transfer. We would need to accept that either London was infected directly from the Continent (quite possible) or that the agent was not reliant on rats and fleas.

A fourth contribution of the London evidence is that, as was first identified by Sam Cohn, the impacts of the four successive plagues under review reduces steadily and markedly. He suggests that some kind of immunity to the pathogen was acquired over a relatively short time. Such immunity would not be characteristic of modern bubonic plague.[563] Cohn argues that the pestilence in Florence broke out not in the zone where the grain store was situated, a recurrent feature of twentieth-century outbreaks in India, but particularly in the impoverished, highly populated quarters of the city.[564] London can advance no definitive evidence on this aspect of the plague since rich and poor lived very much side by side in the city, but there are hints that the pestilence killed the poor more readily.

A comparison of the rates of prevalence of bone lesions (picked up during life prior to contraction of the plague), from which those who were buried at the East Smithfield cemetery suffered, with those from pre-1348 medieval cemetery assemblage, has concluded that once infected, the weaker and less healthy individuals were more likely to succumb to the disease.[565] It seems likely that, in general, poverty would contribute to an increased incidence of such environmental or occupational stresses. Coupled with the fact that the physical stature of those buried at East Smithfield was generally lower than other late medieval cemetery assemblages, this supports a general notion that the poor were more affected than the rich. In her consideration of the squeeze on day-patient care at Westminster Abbey from 1350 onwards, Barbara Harvey speculates that one possible reason may have been that 'those who survived [the plague] were perhaps the fittest who did not have these kinds of needs'.[566]

Therefore, while rats were present in London to act as a potential bubonic go-between, the season and speed of the outbreak would require that the epidemic was either very significantly a pneumonic variant bubonic plague, or was not bubonic plague at all. The apparent and rapid decrease in mortality rates of successive outbreaks after 1349 would suggest the latter. The need for more detailed scientific studies on pre-plague skeletal collections to establish the presence of *Y. pestis* ancient DNA would certainly help inform this debate.

NOTES

1 Translation of the Register of Charterhouse in St John Hope 1925, 7.
2 Benedictow 2004; Cohn 2002.
3 Röhrkasten 2001; Megson 1998.
4 Sharpe 1889, 1890.
5 CHW, Vol. 1, xiv; xxii: The wills related only to property in the city, setting a benchmark for those enrolling them; furthermore, enrolment of each cost 15s 10d – a significant sum in itself.
6 The widest review of the wills is that of Weetman 2004, analysing trends from 1259–1370. Röhrkasten 2001 represents the most detailed review of the evidence for the period from 1348–1400. Other studies have included Cohn 2003, 197; Benedictow 2004, 136.
7 Freemen citizens and their families were a much smaller group than the entire resident population of London; it has been estimated that they made up slightly more than a quarter of the total population (CPMR, Vol. 2, xlvii–liv).
8 Röhrkasten 2001, 176–7; Megson 1998, 129.
9 From 1327–47, an average of twenty-eight wills were drawn up, and 27.2 enrolled per annum, ranging between a minimum of sixteen wills and fifteen enrolments (in 1344) and a maximum of forty-nine wills and fifty-two enrolments (in 1328): CHW, Vol. 1.
10 Estimates for 80,000 by about 1300 are provided in Keene 1984; a lower figure of 60,000 is argued in Nightingale 1996. The famine years of the early fourteenth century saw a national population drop of perhaps 10 to 15 per cent (e.g. Nightingale 2005, 44). The issue of whether the population subsequently rose or remained static between then and 1348 is unclear (Barron 2004, 239). I have elected to assume a population of 60,000 in 1348.

11 Between 1347 and 1375, women were responsible for just 13.8 per cent of all Husting wills, a figure that dropped to 12.1 per cent between 1375 and 1400.

12 Wood 2003.

13 VCH Middx 2, Appendix 1, 102–3.

14 Weetman 2004, 40–51.

15 Röhrkasten 2001, 180.

16 TNA SC 2/191/60.

17 DNB, 2, 378.

18 The disease was known to medieval people as the great mortality, pestilence or epidemic: the term 'Black Death' was not coined until much later.

19 Cohn 2003, 154; Riley 1863, 252; Martin 1996. Knighton was a canon of Leicester Abbey. An epidemic also visited Florence in March to June of 1340, causing many deaths (Henderson 1988, 253). This killed 34 per cent of men, 34 per cent of women and 32 per cent of children, buried by the Company of Roast Chestnuts in the parish of San Frediano.

20 CPMR, Vol. 1, 143–64.

21 Although in 1341 there had been forty-five wills drawn, compared to an average since 1327 of twenty-eight, and a figure of just twenty-one for 1343 itself: CHW, Vol. 1.

22 Tuchmann 1989, 91.

23 Carlin 1996, 143.

24 Blatherwick and Bluer 2009, 60–75.

25 Phillpotts 1999.

26 Rosser 1989, 167–70.

27 Benedictow 2004.

28 Benedictow 2004, 96–109.

29 Hardy 1869, Vol. 1, 361.

30 CPL, Vol. 3, 37–8.

31 Horrox 1994, 221.

32 CPR, Ed III, Vol. 8, 142.

33 Hamilton-Thompson 1914, 102; Horrox 1994, 111–12.

34 Horrox 1994, 112.

35 Horrox 1994, 114.

36 CPR, Ed III, Vol. 8, 147.

37 CPR, Ed III, Vol. 8, 146–7.

38 CPR, Ed III, Vol. 8, 144. The twenty-four 'poor' knights were, of course, the Order of the Garter.

39 Wilson et al. 1986, 82–3.

40 Ashbee 2007, Chapter 7.

41 CPR, Ed III, Vol. 8, 149.

42 CCR, Ed III, Vol. 8, 559.

43 CPR, Ed III, Vol. 8, 151.

44 CCR, Ed III, Vol. 8, 588.

45 CLB F, 183.
46 CPR, Ed III, Vol. 8, 183.
47 Hardy 1869, Vol. 1, 363.
48 CCR, Ed III, Vol. 8, 585.
49 CCR, Ed III, Vol. 8, 588.
50 CAN, DD, no 416.
51 CAN, DD, no 417.
52 CHW, Vol. 1, 505–632.
53 CPL, Vol. 3, 286, 310.
54 TNA SC 2/191/60.
55 Infectious diseases have an incubation stage and an infectious stage; the duration of these may vary from hours to weeks. For a short review of the debates over the nature of the plague, and how the London evidence can contribute, see the Appendix.
56 See Appendix. This proposition would clearly mean a later arrival and faster spread. If it is right, there is no obvious explanation for the number of chroniclers setting the date as July or August for the plague's arrival. It remains the case that the combined evidence of discrete manorial courts and Episcopal institutions provides a sounder basis for analysis than chronicles.
57 Hardy 1869, Vol. 1, 359.
58 Horrox 1984, 250.
59 TNA E 403/345 m1 (payment is dated Wednesday 1 October 1348). Perhaps a scribal error is to blame.
60 Horrox 1994, 113–14; Philip Ziegler (1977, 122 n5) referenced this erroneously as evidence that London was already being ravaged by this date.
61 Horrox 115; Parry 1912, 137.
62 Giles 1847, 189; Horrox 1994, 81; Luard 1866, 475.
63 CHW, Vol. 1, 506–7.
64 TNA SC 2/191/60 m1–2.
65 Johnson 1948, Vol. 2; CCRBL, 134 (l).
66 CLB F, 185.
67 Foedera, Vol. 5, 643, 646.
68 CPR, Ed III, Vol. 8, 193.
69 CPR, Ed III, Vol. 8, 202.
70 Horrox 1994, 115–16.
71 Duffy 1992, 293.
72 Barron 2004, 330.
73 CPL, Vol. 3, 272.
74 Thompson 1889, 406–7; Horrox 1994, 65.
75 CPL, Vol. 3, 309.
76 Foedera, Vol. 5, 649.
77 Mortimer 2008, 262.

78　CCR, Ed III, Vol. 8, 606–7.

79　Gentleman's Magazine, Vol. 1 (new series), 1834, January–June, 217; the location in the retro-choir of the slab is discussed in Divers et al. 2009, 67, monument L438. I am grateful to Nathalie Cohen for drawing my attention to this work.

80　CHW, Vol. 1, 518, 526, 609.

81　CLB F, 185.

82　TNA SC 2/191/60 m4.

83　Hockey 1987, 25.

84　Horrox 1994, 74.

85　Horrox 1994, 22–3.

86　Horrox 1994, 81.

87　Horrox 1994, 64, 74, 81.

88　Horrox 1994, 28–30.

89　Horrox 1994, 194–203.

90　Horrox 1994, 52–3.

91　Hurston 1856. The original document is lost and undated, however, so could as easily refer to the 1361 or even later outbreaks.

92　VCH Middx 2, 61–70.

93　Hockey 1986, nos 331–2, 345, 354, 363. The dates of institution, often several weeks later than the vacancies themselves, were recorded in the register on 22 and 14 January, and 2, 15 and 20 February respectively.

94　TNA SC 2/205/12 m9d.

95　CHW, Vol. 1, 608.

96　CPR, Ed III, Vol. 8, 177–9.

97　Horrox 194, 81; Bernard d'Espaygne, a wine merchant, was beheaded at Nomanneslond in 1326 for treason (Riley 1863, 266); BL Ms Nero E vi; MOSJ MS K/12, 28.

98　Kingsford 1908, Vol. 2, 81–2.

99　So named in the Cartulary of the Knights Hospitaller; BL Ms Nero E vi; MOSJ MS K/12, p. 36, charter dated to 1432.

100　Tyler 1998, 118–19, fig. 5.

101　Horrox 1994, 64–5.

102　Horrox 1994, 53.

103　Harvey 1993, 115–16.

104　CCR, Ed III, Vol. 8, 615; Horrox 1994, 71.

105　Foedera, Vol. 5, 655.

106　Mortimer 2008, 262.

107　Ziegler 1977, 72–5; Riley 1868, 264–5.

108　Horrox 1994, 74, quoting John of Reading.

109　CPL, Vol. 3, Gilbert Palmer and his wife Alice, and William Blod and his wife Joan.

110　CHW, Vol. 1, 518, 524–5, 528–30, 571, 640–1, 647, 661.

111 CHW, Vol. 1, 600; 602.

112 CHW, Vol. 1, 517.

113 CHW, Vol. 1, 514, 519.

114 CHW, Vol. 1, 515.

115 CPR, Ed III, Vol. 8, 218, 254; CHW, Vol. 1, 512; Hockey 1986 (ed.), no 404.

116 TNA SC 2/191/60 m6–m12d.

117 Horrox 1994, 32.

118 TNA LR 2/61, translated by W. St John Hope 1925, 7–8.

119 Levillain 2002, 1, 221.

120 *Oxford Dictionary of National Biography*: www.oxforddnb.com/index/17/101017985/; CPR, Ed III, Vol. 8, 332.

121 St John Hope 1925, 7–8; Pugh 1969, 159.

122 CPP, Vol. 22, 234.

123 St John Hope 1925, 7.

124 CPR, Ed III, Vol. 8, 266.

125 Horrox 1994, 81.

126 Horrox 1994, 65; a garbling of this has led to a miscalculation of 2,000 burials in one cemetery between 2 February and 2 April 1348 (Gottfried 1983, 64; Naphy and Spicer 2004, 31).

127 Horrox 1994, 70, quoting the *Historia Roffensis* attributed to William of Dene.

128 Barber and Thomas 2002, 13–14.

129 PRO C 54 185 m27, translated by Dr Jeremy Ashbee.

130 CLPA, nos 65, 68. This should be placed in the context of twenty-four such alleged violent dispossessions between 1340 and 1450 (with breaks in the sequence).

131 CLB F, 203.

132 CLB G, 30–31.

133 TNA SC 2/191/60 m9–m12d; SC 2/205/12 m10.

134 CCR, Ed III, Vol. 9, 8–9.

135 CCR, Ed III, Vol. 9, 54. The search encompassed many other English ports, too.

136 MOSJ MS K/12, Baildon transcript of Cotton MS Nero E vi, fo 15d.

137 LMA Husting Rolls 77/49, 77/126 (information courtesy of Tony Dyson, Nick Holder and Nathalie Cohen).

138 CHW, Vol. 1, 534, 537.

139 TNA SC 2/191/60 esp m13–m15d; Riley 1868, liii.

140 TNA SC 2/191/60 m21; CHW, Vol. 1, 535.

141 CHW, Vol. 1, 531–2.

142 CHW, Vol. 1, 556.

143 CHW, Vol. 1, 558; detail of will transcribed from microfilm at LMA by Dr Jeremy Ashbee.

144 St John Hope 1925, 7.

145 Grimes 1968, 175–80.

146 CPR, Ed III, Vol. 8, 331; CAN, no 437; Grainger and Phillpotts 2011, 75; TNA E 40/2643.

147 Hodgett 1971, no 951.

148 Hodgett 1971, no 958.

149 CHW, Vol. 1, 651, 679; detail transcribed from LMA microfiche by Dr Jeremy Ashbee.

150 TNA E 210/6811.

151 TNA E 326/2310.

152 CHW, Vol. 1, 597.

153 Foedera, Vol. 5, 658, transcribed by Dr Jeremy Ashbee.

154 IPM, Ed III, Vol. 9, nos 368, 428.

155 CPR, Ed III, Vol. 8, 261.

156 CPR, Ed III, Vol. 8, 271.

157 CCR, Ed III, Vol. 9, 62–4.

158 CPMR, Vol. 1, 224.

159 CLB F, 191.

160 CLB F, 186.

161 CHW, Vol. 1, 567, 581, 599; Hist Gaz, St Pancras Soper Lane no 145/36.

162 Her guardianship was assigned on 13 June 1353 to Thomas de Staundone, cofferer, and she claimed her property at full age in 1362 (CLB G, 8, 145).

163 CHW, Vol. 1, 558, 576.

164 CHW, Vol. 1, 543, 563.

165 CLB F, 189.

166 CHW, Vol. 1, 598.

167 CLB G, 11–12; CAD, C 6871.

168 CHW, Vol. 1, 552.

169 CHW, Vol. 1, 562–3.

170 Barron 1985, 23–5.

171 CHW, Vol. 1, 540, 542, 547, 565, 679; see Chapter 5 for further consideration of fraternities.

172 CPR, Ed III, Vol. 4, 105.

173 CHW, Vol. 1, 552; CPL, Vol. 3, 289.

174 CHW, Vol. 1, 675.

175 CHW, Vol. 1, 544, 590; see also Redstone and Redstone 1937.

176 CHW, Vol. 1, 618, 619.

177 Westlake 1923, Vol. 1, 110.

178 CPL, Vol. 3, 274.

179 CHW, Vol. 1, 569.

180 TNA LR 15/163.

181 CAD, Vol. 4 (1902), A 7378.

182 CLB F, 221.

183 TNA SC 2/191/60 m16–m19d.

184 CHW, Vol. 1, 652.

185 CPR, Ed III, Vol. 8, 277.

186 CCR, Ed III, Vol. 9, 65.

187 CHW, Vol. 1, 564.

188 TNA SC 2/191/60 m16d.

189 CHW, Vol. 1, 569; CLB F, 188, 191.

190 CLB F, 191.

191 Jones 1964, 20–2.

192 Horrox 1994, 64–5, after Thompson 1889, 406–7.

193 Sporley's *History of the abbots of Westminster*, written *c.* 1450 (BL Cotton MS Claud A viii), quoted by Dugdale, 1817, Monasticon, Vol. 1, 275, translated by Dr Jeremy Ashbee.

194 Cal Hust Wills, Vol. 1, 578.

195 CPR, Ed III, Vol. 8, 285, 286. Reasons for vacancy could include death, resignation, exchange or cessation; dates of presentation to a vacant benefice could be anywhere from a few days to several weeks after vacancy. Actual institution might follow days, weeks or months after the presentation (see Aberth 1995). The dates here suggest deaths in April or May.

196 CPR, Ed III, Vol. 8, 285, 291.

197 CPR, Ed III, Vol. 8, 287; CHW, Vol. 1, 559.

198 CPL, Vol. 3, 273–4.

199 CPL, Vol. 3, 285.

200 CPL, Vol. 3, 330; CPP, Vol. 1, 165.

201 VCH London 1, 542–6; CPR, Ed III, Vol. 8, 348.

202 CHW, Vol. 1, 568, 580, 595.

203 Harvey 2000, 18, quoting WAM 19331; John of Reading is described as '*tunc infirmario*' ('then the infirmarer') on 15 March 1350, presumably appointed following the death of John de Ryngestede during the plague.

204 Ahl 2002, 18–19.

205 CHW, Vol. 1, 586; Kingsford 1915, 101.

206 CHW, Vol. 1, 571.

207 TNA SC 2/191/60 m20–m22d.

208 CPR, Ed III, Vol. 8, 295, 298.

209 CAN, no 617: the complaint was brought following the reconstruction of the forge in May 1377.

210 CFR, Ed III, Vol. 6; CHW, Vol. 1, 577.

211 CPMR, Vol. 1, A6, m1b.

212 CAN, Roll DD, no 418. Hardyngham was litigious, see note 50.

213 Sutton 2005, 96.

214 Pugh 1968, 280.

215 TNA E 101 471/3, translated by Dr Jeremy Ashbee.

216 Gask 1926, 15.

217 CPR, Ed III, Vol. 8, 298.

218 Foedera, Vol. 5, 662, transcribed by Dr Jeremy Ashbee.

219 CLPA, no 67.

220 CHW, Vol. 1, 691; Vol. 2, 70.

221 CHW, Vol. 1, ix.

222 CHW, Vol. 1, 603, 649–51.

223 CCR, Vol. 9, 163.

224 Barron 2004, 39.

225 CFR, Ed III, Vol. 6, 140; CPR, Ed III, Vol. 8, 303.

226 CPR, Ed III, Vol. 8, 309, 332.

227 CPR, Ed III, Vol. 8, 305.

228 CLB F, 192.

229 CLB F, 192; Horrox 1994, 287–9.

230 CLB F, 192.

231 CPMR, Vol. 1, A6, m1b.

232 CLB G, ix.

233 CHW, Vol. 1, 608, 610; Vol. 2, 80.

234 CHW, Vol. 1, 607.

235 CHW, Vol. 1, 607–8.

236 CHW, Vol. 1, 600, 602.

237 CPR, Ed III, Vol. 8, 347, 354.

238 CPR, Ed III, Vol. 8, 388, 355.

239 Ormrod 1989, 856.

240 TNA SC 2/191/61 m20–24d.

241 CHW, Vol. 1, 641.

242 Riley 1868, 244–7.

243 CPR, Ed III, Vol. 8, 389.

244 CHW, Vol. 1, 567; CLB F, 193.

245 CLB F, 216; CHW, Vol. 1, 596.

246 CPMR, Vol. 1, A6, m2; CLB F, 199.

247 CPMR, Vol. 1, A6, m2b. This had a happy ending since on 13 April 1372,
     'Juliana, daughter of John Sellyng, acknowledged a loan of £3 2s 4d from
     John Lytlyngton, to be repaid out of 100s rents assigned to her by William
     de Stoke, tailor, that amount being in the latter's keeping as her guardian'
     (CPMR, Vol. 2, A17, m4b).

248 CHW, Vol. 1, 512, 524; CLB G, 57. De Northerne could not be found, so
     his properties and goods were seized.

249 CLB F, 207; CHW, Vol. 1, 535, 616.

250 Horrox 1994, 72.

251 CIPM, Ed III, Vol. 9, 302.

252 CPL, Vol. 3, 327.

253 Naphy and Spicer (2004, 32), following Gottfried (1983, 64), claim that
     290 deaths per day were recorded between June and September 1349, but
     no basis for this figure has been found.

254 Horrox 1994, 153–4.

255 CPL,Vol. 3, 42.

256 CHW,Vol. 1, ix: the court was suspended for harvest time, and this clearly included the whole of August and September each year.

257 CHW,Vol. 1, 608–9, 611, 614, 618.

258 CHW,Vol. 1, 616; CPR, Ed III,Vol. 8, 455.

259 CLB F, 110.

260 Röhrkasten 2001, 189.

261 CLPA, nos 66–68.

262 CLPA, no 57.

263 CHW,Vol. 1, 555, 572, 621–2.

264 Luard 1866, 412.

265 CLB F, 199.

266 CPMR,Vol. 1, A6, m3b.

267 CLB F, 199.

268 CPR, Ed III,Vol. 8, 459; CLB F, 210.

269 Horrox 1994, 118.

270 CHW,Vol. 1, 626.

271 CHW,Vol. 1, 625. Richard survived until 1363 but his little sister is not mentioned in his will (CHW,Vol. 2, 77).

272 TNA E 101/472, translated and summarised by Dr Jeremy Ashbee.

273 St Paul's by 1345, Salisbury Cathedral by February 1349 and Hereford by July 1349: CPL,Vol. 3, 184, 293, 319.

274 Sharpe 1885, 9.

275 Riley 1868, 251–2. De Hethe was apparently afterwards imprisoned for impersonating the Pope's secretary. Though pardoned in 1352 by the king, he was again accused of impersonation four years later, his role this time that of a canon of Hereford Cathedral (Parry 1912, 244).

276 TNA E 40/2645; CPR, Ed III,Vol. 8, 484.

277 Platt 1997 (3rd imp.), 6.

278 The averaged figure is consistent with the results from the *pestis secunda*, where the average from seven individuals (about 5 per cent of the sample) indicates death at a point 27 per cent of the way through the same period.

279 I am very grateful to Penny Tucker for sharing her analysis of the Husting court sessions with me.

280 TNA CP 40. I am very grateful to Graham Dawson for sharing his preliminary evidence with me.

281 Barber and Thomas 2002, 12–13; Museum of London Archaeology Service unpublished evaluation report site code GLY01.

282 Grainger et al. 2008, 12.

283 The provision of age and sex to any individual skeleton is not 100 per cent certain (e.g. Chamberlain 2006); demographic data are derived from the Centre for Human Bioarchaeology database at the Museum of London

and have been grouped into cohorts and matched to archaeological evidence by the author as part of a study on medieval monastic cemeteries: http://ads.ahds.ac.uk/catalogue/archive/cemeteries_ahrb_2005/index. cfm?CFID=31460&CFTOKEN=63267820

284 S.N. DeWitte, 2007 (data from 490 specimens generously supplied by DeWitte and converted into age/sex categories as used in Table 3a/3b).

285 Grainger et al. 2008, 33.

286 Hatcher 1986, 31.

287 Grainger et al. 2008, 55.

288 CLB G, 15.

289 See, for example, Gottfried 1980, 9: London's tax returns for 1377 indicate a ratio of men to women of 1.07:1.

290 Hollingsworth and Hollingsworth 1971; though this is not true of all episodes of plague analysed: see S. Ell 1985.

291 Lomas 1989, 130.

292 Laurent 1937, nos 730–865.

293 Evans in prep; the burials were dated, by dendrochronology of the remarkably well-preserved coffins, to 1349 in several instances.

294 For a discussion of this issue, see Gilchrist and Sloane 2005, Chapter 5.2.

295 Gilchrist and Sloane 2005, Table 7.

296 Hawkins 1990, 641, for putrefaction; Gilchrist and Sloane 2005, Chapter 5.2; Gilchrist 2008, 144–7.

297 Gilchrist and Sloane 2005, 102.

298 Horrox 1994, 31–2.

299 Dohar 1995, 39.

300 Lütgert 2000, 258.

301 Horrox 1994, 268–9.

302 C. Thomas, personal communication.

303 Ziegler 1969 (1997 edn), 124; Naphy and Spicer 2004, 31; Olea and Christakos 2005, 299–300.

304 Britnell 1994, 198–9; Röhrkasten 2004, 77.

305 See Nightingale 2005, 40–1.

306 Megson 1998.

307 Hovland 2006, 208–9.

308 Hennessey, 1898. I have also included evidence from the Husting wills which augments Hennessey's original work.

309 CPP, 234, 395.

310 CPP, 468.

311 St John Hope, 25, 7–8; Kingsford 1908, II, 81–2.

312 TNA E 328/6.

313 Hawkins 1990, 642.

314 CLB G, 85.

315 Riley 1868, 264–5.

316 VCH Middx 5, 49–55.

317 Karlsson 1996, 271, quoting *Islandske Annaler indtil 1578*.

318 CHW; Thrupp 1996.

319 Oxford: Salter 1912, 29–59; Colchester: Benham 1907, 55–9; Lincoln: Hill 1948, 251–2; York and Norwich: Dunn 2003, 32–3; for an overview, Britnell 1994.

320 Britnell 1994, 200.

321 Lomas 1989, 129.

322 Hatcher 1994, 9.

323 Dyer 1980, 237–8; Arthur 2005, 120; Ecclestone 1999.

324 CIPM, 176, 190, 202, 204, 222, 230, 390, 664.

325 Givry: Benedictow 2004, 105; Orvieto: Cohn 2003, 171; Siena and San Gimignano: Bowsky 1964, 11, 17; Perpignan: Emery 1967, 616.

326 PROME, II, 225, m6.

327 PROME, II, 224, m4.

328 PROME, II, 231, m2.

329 Lindley 1996 (2003), 139.

330 PROME, II, 227, m4; Horrox 1994, 312–4.

331 Putnam 1908, 136–7; CLB G, 115–8.

332 Beveridge 1955, 20; table 1. Costs based on 'decadal' averages 1340–8 and 1349–59.

333 Beveridge 1955, tables 3 and 4.

334 Harvey 1993, 172–3; Shaw 2000, 190.

335 Hatcher 1994, 7; Munro 2004, 8–9.

336 Galloway 2000, 31, 42.

337 PROME, II, 260, m32.

338 Nightingale 2005, 46–7.

339 Glovers by 6 January 1350; shearmen by 15 February 1350; furbishers by 5 July 1350 (CLB F).

340 CPMR, Vol. 1, A6 (pp. 224–40), m7.

341 Putnam 1915, 23; Dohar 2000, 187.

342 William Langland, Piers Plowman: *The Prologue*, lines 80–3. For a discussion on resignation rates in the diocese of Ely during the pestilence, see Aberth 1995, 281–3.

343 Putnam 1908, 91.

344 Logan 1996, reviewed by B. Harvey in *J Eccles Hist.*, Vol. 49, No 1, January 1998, 171–2.

345 Westlake 1923, Vol. 1, 110; Vol. 2, 395; WAM 50698; there were twenty-eight monks and the abbot in 1381 according to the poll tax collected in that year.

346 Harvey 2000, esp. 20–2.

347 Westlake 1923, Vol. 2, 297, 341.

348 For the Eleanor dole, see Harvey 1993, 27–8; for the abbey almonry, see Rushton 2002, esp. 77.

349 Röhrkasten 2004, 77, 79–80; Kingsford 1915, 62.

350 TNA E 143/9/14.

351 CLB G, 28; CPL 3, 574–5.

352 CLB G, 43, 49–50; Sabine 1933, 343.

353 Riley 1868, 295–300.

354 Hanawalt 1993, 48.

355 Hanawalt 1993, 57.

356 Thrupp 1996, 203.

357 CHW, Vol. 2, 664, 695.

358 Röhrkasten 2001, 190.

359 Axworthy 2000, 301.

360 Norris 1991, 186–7; Badham 2000, 232.

361 Lindley 2003, 130–1.

362 Martin 1996, 184.

363 Gairdner 1876, 67–88.

364 Galbraith 1927, 50.

365 Gransden 1957, 275.

366 CHW, Vol. 2, 13.

367 Britnell nd, no 59.

368 Gransden 1957, 275.

369 Horrox 1994, 85–6.

370 Horrox 1994, 86.

371 Röhrkasten 2001, 192.

372 CLB H, 17.

373 CHW, Vol. 2, 17, 26, 18.

374 Hardy 1869, 417.

375 CHW, Vol. 2, 27.

376 St John Hope 1925, 9–10.

377 TNA E 326/2315.

378 CPR, Ed III, Vol. 12, 2.

379 CPR Ed III, Vol. 11, 567.

380 CPR Ed III, Vol. 12, 20.

381 CCR, Ed III, Vol. 11, 248.

382 CLB G, 134–5.

383 CHW, Vol. 2, 60–1, 22, 49.

384 CHW, Vol. 2, 19; CLB G, 122.

385 CPR, Ed III, Vol. 12, 176; CHW, Vol. 2, 22, 37.

386 CCR, Ed III, Vol. 9, 181–2.

387 Rickert 1952.

388 CFR, Vol. 7, 158; CPR, Ed III, Vol. 12, 21, 19.

389 Carlin 1996, 286; VCH London 1, 542.

390 CPR, Ed III, Vol. 12, 22, 39.

391 CHW, Vol. 2, 31.

392 Harvey 1993, 84; Harvey 2000, 18 n35; CLB G, 129.

393 CHW, Vol. 2, 299; CLB G, 128.

394 CAD, Vol. 6, C 6385.

395 Harvey 1947; CHW, Vol. 2, 106.

396 CHW, Vol. 2, 26.

397 CHW, Vol. 2, 23 (qv CHW, Vol. 1, 572).

398 CHW, Vol. 2, 24.

399 CPR, Ed III, Vol. 12, 25.

400 CPR, Ed III, Vol. 12, 42, 80; CHW, Vol. 2, 30, 73.

401 CPR, Ed III, Vol. 12, 73.

402 Tytler 1845, 36; Reid 1928, 122.

403 CPR, Ed III, Vol. 12, 36; CHW, Vol. 2, 38.

404 Cohn 2003, 143.

405 CPR, Ed III, Vol. 4, 441; Vol. 10, 288; Vol. 13, 194; CCR, Ed III, 291; CHW, Vol. 2, 56.

406 CCR, Ed III, Vol. 9, 197–8.

407 Horrox 1994, 119.

408 CHW, Vol. 2, 44.

409 CHW, Vol. 2, 59–60.

410 CPR, Ed III, Vol. 12, 53; Fasti, Vol. 5, 66–8.

411 CPR, Ed III, Vol. 12, 61–2.

412 CAD, Vol. 2, A 2686.

413 CHW, Vol. 2, 24; CAD, Vol. 5, A 11790.

414 CHW, Vol. 2, 33.

415 CLB G, 133.

416 CHW, Vol. 2, 46; CPR, Ed III, Vol. 14, 178–9.

417 TNA C 241/141/128; CHW, Vol. 2, 61, 63.

418 Carlin 1996, 286; VCH London 1, 538–42; VCH Middx 1, 193–204; Harvey 1993, 102; 116 n12; McHardy 1977, 29–38.

419 CCR, Ed III, Vol. 9, 370.

420 CPR, Ed III, Vol. 9, 488.

421 Grainger et al. 2008, 30.

422 TNA E 42/447; CHW, Vol. 2, 90.

423 CCR, 1422–27, 211; TNA SC 6/917/16.

424 At 95 per cent confidence rating. The cemetery went out of use in 1539 so the burial dates to between 1402 and 1539.

425 Gilchrist and Sloane 2005, Chapter 8.

426 Bolton 1996, 27; Naphy and Spicer 2004, 34.

427 Megson 1998, 133.

428 CHW, Vol. 1, 608.

429 Horrox 1994, 88; Gransden 1957, 277.

430 Exceptions are Bridbury 1973, 584; Röhrkasten 2001.

431 Cohn 2003, 197; Giles 1845, 173.

432 Fitch 1979.

433 Röhrkasten 2001, 196, implying approximately 10 per cent mortality during the plague.

434 CHW, Vol. 2, 109, 115, 131; Fitch 1979, 398, 424.

435 Ormrod 1996, 150.

436 CAN, nos 538–44.

437 CLB G, 226.

438 CLB G, 228.

439 CLB G, 230.

440 CLB G, 229. I thank Dr Claire Martin for the explanation of this type of guardianship.

441 CPR, Ed III, Vol. 14, 272.

442 CHW, Vol. 2, 117, 122; Fitch 1979, 178.

443 CAD, Vol. 2, A 1927.

444 Duncan nd, book 25.

445 CPMR, Vol. 2, A13, 84–95.

446 CHW, Vol. 2, 112, 129.

447 Röhrkasten 2001, 192.

448 CHW, Vol. 2, 125, transcribed by Dr Jeremy Ashbee.

449 CHW, Vol. 2, 120; CPMR, A14, m2.

450 Davis 1993, 56; BL MS Nero E vi, fo 4d.

451 Horrox 1994, 88.

452 Röhrkasten 2001, 198.

453 CHW, Vol. 2, 171, 173, 187.

454 Röhrkasten 2001, 198.

455 CHW, Vol. 2, 174.

456 CPMR, Vol. 2, A21, m5.

457 Röhrkasten 2001, 198.

458 CHW, Vol. 2, 175, 181.

459 John de Norwich does not appear in lists of masters of the hospital in the Victoria County History, or as updated by Barron and Davies. He first appears in 1354 when his estate was ratified by the king (CPR, Ed III, Vol. 10, 74), so he must have replaced William Weston in 1352 or 1353, and his successor was recognised in 1376 (CAD, Vol. 2, A 2334); therefore, he ran the hospital for over twenty-two years.

460 CPR, Ed III, Vol. 16, 159.

461 Horrox 1994, 120.

462 CPMR, Vol. 2, 199.

463 CHW, Vol. 2, 225; Harvey 1993, 76.v.

464 Röhrkasten 2001, 199–200.

465 Riley 1868, 384.

466 Röhrkasten 2001, 199–200.

467 1377 London and Middlesex Poll Tax: Fenwick 2001 (pt 2), 61–2;

Southwark: Carlin 1996, 142–3; Westminster: Rosser 1989, 162; adult population estimates for London: Russell 1948, 285–7.

468 Nightingale 1995, 239.

469 Hanawalt 2007, 27–8; Carlin 1996, 139; Megson 1996, 25; Gottfried 1980, 9; Goldberg 1990, 212–3.

470 Nightingale 1995, 208.

471 Holt 1987, 205–6.

472 Dunn 2003, 33.

473 Gooder 1998, 40–3; VCH Oxford 4, 3–73.

474 Martin 1996, 105.

475 Keene 1990, 30–8.

476 O'Connor 1993, 63, 101–2; Schofield 1995, 55; Carlin 1996, 46–7; Rosser 1989, 68–73.

477 Ormrod 1996; Braid in prep; Haddock and Kielsing 2002.

478 Riley 1861, 4.

479 Riley 1861, 29.

480 Cohn 2002, 38–9; Thrupp 1996, 201–6.

481 Hovland 2006, 174.

482 Hovland 2006, 81: the sums rose again to 6s 6d in 1418.

483 Hovland 2006, 51, 136.

484 Braid in prep.

485 Hovland 2006, 229, 239.

486 Badham 2000, 232.

487 Blackmore and Pearce 2010, 20.

488 Riley 1868, 267; CLBF, 241.

489 Horrox 1994, 131–4.

490 Riley 1868, 319; Ipswich had one: Twiss 1873, 164–5.

491 CLBF, 208; CHW, Vol. 2, 114.

492 CLBG, 78, 169, 192, 295; Riley 1861, 508.

493 Rushton 2002.

494 See Chapter 3.

495 For London dormitories, see, for example, Schofield and Lea 2005, 125; Sloane and Malcolm 2004, 92; for hospital and infirmary halls, see, for example, Orme and Webster 1995, 90–1; Prescott 1992, 38–41.

496 Miller and Saxby 2007, 86–7, 126; Harvey and Oeppen 2001, 222.

497 Harvey and Oeppen 2001, 227–30, 233.

498 Weetman 2004, 143, 146, 173, chart 4c; CHW, Vol. 2, 18, 39, 106.

499 CCRC, 61.

500 Thompson 1965, 186.

501 Barron 1985; Weetman 2004, 171.

502 Calculated from an analysis of the Husting wills by the author.

503 Barron 1985, 25.

504 CHW, Vol. 1, 482, 637; Vol. 2, 106, 147, 218.

505 Riley 1868, 230, 365, 384, 388.

506 Rawcliffe 2006, 282–3.

507 Rawcliffe 2006, 109.

508 Rawcliffe 2006, 13–47.

509 Carlin 1996, 103–4.

510 CLB K, 124–6; CCR 40–270.

511 Thompson 1965, 185.

512 CHW, Vol. 2, 283.

513 CHW, Vols 1 and 2; this cannot take account of the missing roll for 1360.

514 Weetman 2004, 232.

515 Harding 1992, 126.

516 CHW, Vol. 2, 187.

517 Wood-Legh 1932, 50; Kreider 1979, 72; Rousseau 2003, 27–30; Boldrick 1997, 26.

518 Weetman 2004, 89–104; CHW, Vol. 1, 665.

519 Gilchrist and Sloane 2005, 94; Gilchrist 2008.

520 There are a number of works which summarise the debates, including Theilmann and Cate, 2007, and especially Nutton 2008.

521 Benedictow 2004, Chapter 3: a flea biting an infected rat develops a plug of multiplying bacteria blocking its stomach. Starving, it regurgitates parts of the bacterial block as it tries to feed, introducing the disease into the bloodstream of its host. As starving fleas transfer to new rat hosts, the colony suffers an epizootic. As the rats die, the fleas are forced to attack new hosts including humans, introducing the plague to them.

522 Cohn 2003, 8.

523 Benedictow 2004, 20.

524 For bubonic outbreaks, Cohn (2003, 19) quotes 2.68 per cent for Bombay City in 1903; Benedictow (2004, 31) tabulates an overall mortality rate for the Bombay Presidency of 2.38 per cent in 1897–8, but with local figures up to 36 per cent in smaller settlements such as Ibrampur. Thielman and Cate (2007, 385) quote similar ranges from three Manchurian outbreaks in 1910–21 of 2 per cent up to 25 per cent in some villages.

525 Temperatures between 18°C and 27°C and a relative humidity of 70 per cent are ideal, whereas temperatures below 7°C are deleterious to all developmental stages except the adult, Duncan and Scott 2005, 316.

526 For example, Horrox 2006; Wray 2004.

527 Drancourt et al. 1998; Raoult et al. 2000; Wood and DeWitte-Avina 2003; Prentice et al. 2004; Thomas et al. 2004; Drancourt et al. 2007; Haensch et al. 2010.

528 Gasquet 1893, 7–8.

529 Bean 1963, 426.

530 Shrewsbury 1970, 3, 6.

531 Ell 1979.

532 Siraisi 1982, 11. Siraisi was concerned about the capacity for bacteria to mutate.

533 Twigg 1984; reviewed by Wilkinson 1985; Gottfried 1986; Palmer 1987.

534 Bean 1982, 26–7.

535 Davis 1986; Audoin-Rouzeau 1999; McCormick 2003.

536 Karlsson 1996; Steffensen 1974.

537 Scott and Duncan 2001; 2004.

538 For example, http://scienceblogs.com/aetiology/2008/01/did_yersinia_pestis_really_cau_1.php. For a pro-bubonic review of Scott and Duncan by the director of the King's Centre for Military Health Research at King's College London, see www.guardian.co.uk/books/2004/aug/14/features-reviews.guardianreview

539 Cohn 2002; 2003.

540 Wood et al. 2003.

541 Baillie 2006.

542 Eisen et al. 2006.

543 Given-Wilson 2004, 1–20.

544 For example, Benedictow (1994, 128) bases much on the dates; Ziegler (1969, 92–3) is far more circumspect; Shrewsbury (1970, 38) is non-committal.

545 Gasquet 1893, 78; Hamilton-Thompson 1911, 316–7; Benedictow 2004, 124.

546 Davis 1989; Woods et al. 2003, 437–41.

547 WSA D 1/2/3; Fletcher 1922, 1–14.

548 Fletcher, 1922, 6–7; Dorchester (9 miles north of Weymouth) replaced an incumbent on 19 October as did Wool. Blandford, Sturminster Newton and Salisbury (22, 30 and 50 miles north/north-east of Weymouth respectively) replaced clergy between 20 and 28 October.

549 Dorchester: CPR, Ed III, Vol. 8, 185; Bincombe: CPR, Ed III, Vol. 8, 182; Bradford: CPR, Ed III, Vol. 8, 186; Tolpuddle and Piddlehinton (Hynpudel): CPR, Ed III, Vol. 8, 198; Portesham, Abbotsbury, Wareham and Owermoigne (Ogres): CPR, Ed III, Vol. 8, 202–3.

550 Dr Mark Forrest, personal communication.

551 Chanter 1910, 92–8.

552 Rees 1923, 29; Benedictow 2004, 128. Rees references CIPM, Ed III, Vol. 9, no 104 which does not mention pestilence. The only relevant reference is no 353, the inquisition into the holdings of Andrew Braunche held in Frome on 12 August 1349.

553 Shrewsbury 1970, 57; CFR, Ed III, Vol. 6, 182, 198; Bere Regis and Charminster lie between 10 and 20 miles north/north-east of Weymouth.

554 If the pestilence had begun to kill in early September, it must have actually made (invisible) landfall some time earlier. Benedictow (2004, 124) argues sixteen to twenty-three days (for bubonic plague), Scott and Duncan (2005, 162) suggest thirty-two days (haemorrhagic plague), before symptoms

manifest. This would put its biological landfall (*not* its outward recognition) at around early or mid-August.

555 Bowsher et al. 2007, Vol. 1, 155; CD Table 5; CD Table 22.

556 Thomas et al. 2006, 92.

557 Armitage 2001, 85; Liddle 2007.

558 Ainsley 2001, 132; Twigg 1984, 80; Pipe 2007, 88, 95.

559 Wilson 2005, 141; Jones et al. 1985, 604; Ayres and Serjeantson 2002, 170.

560 Shrewsbury 1970, 35; see also Cohn 2003, 30 for a refutation of this theory.

561 Baillie 2006, 34–9; Hallam 1984, 128.

562 Benedictow 2004, 135–77.

563 Cohn 2003, 192; fig. 8.8.

564 Cohn 2003, 205–7.

565 DeWitte and Woods 2008.

566 Harvey 2000, 22.

BIBLIOGRAPHY

Aberth, J., 1995: 'The Black Death in the Diocese of Ely: the evidence of the bishop's register', *Journal of Medieval History*, 21, 275–287

Ahl, D.C., 2002: 'The Misericordia Polyptych: reflections on spiritual and visual culture in Sansepolcro', in Wood, J.M. (ed.), *The Cambridge Companion to Piera della Francesca*, 14–29

Ainsley, C., 2001: 'Animal Bone', in Brigham, T. and Woodger, A., *Roman and Medieval Townhouses on the London Waterfront: Excavations at Governor's House*, City of London (MoLAS Monograph 9)

Armitage, P.L., 2001: 'Mammal, Bird and Fish Bones', in Butler, J., *The City Defences at Aldersgate*, Transactions of the London and Middlesex Archaeological Society, 52, 78–94

Arthur, P., 2005: *The Impact of the Black Death on Seventeen Units of Account of the Bishopric of Winchester* (PhD Winchester University College, University of Southampton)

Ashbee, J., 2007: *The Tower of London as a Royal Residence 1066–1400* (PhD Courtauld Institute, University of London)

Audoin-Rouzeau, F., 1999: 'Le rat noir (Rattus rattus) et la peste dans l'Occident antique et medieval', *Bulletin de la Société de Pathologie Exotique et des ses filiales*, 92, 422–6

Axworthy, R.L., 2000: *The Financial Relationship of the London Merchant Community with Edward III, 1327 to 1377* (PhD Department of History, Royal Holloway, University of London)

Ayres, K. and Serjeantson, D., 2002: 'The Animal Bones', in Allen, T.G. and Hiller, J., *The Excavation of a Medieval Manor House of the Bishops of Winchester at Mount*

House, Witney, Oxfordshire (Oxford Archaeology, Thames Valley landscapes monograph 13), 169–80

Badham, S., 2000: 'Monumental Brasses and the Black Death – A Reappraisal', *Antiquities Journal*, 80, 207–47

Bailey, M., 1996: 'Demographic Decline in Late Medieval England: some thoughts on recent research', *Economic History Review*, ns 49 (1), 1–19

Baillie, M., 2006: *New Light on the Black Death: the cosmic connection* (Stroud)

Barber, B. and Thomas, C., 2002: *The London Charterhouse* (MoLAS Monograph 10) (London)

Barron, C.M., 1985: 'The Parish Fraternities of Medieval London', in Barron, C.M. and Harper-Bill, C., *The Church in Pre-reformation Society*, essays in honour of F.R.H. Du Boulay, 13–37

——, 2004: *London in the Later Middle Ages: Government and People 1200–1500* (Oxford)

Bean, J.M.W., 1963: 'Plague, Population and Economic Decline in England in the Later Middle Ages', *Economic History Review*, ns 15 (3), 423–37

——, 1982: 'The Black Death: The Crisis and its Social and Economic Consequences', in William, D. (ed.), *The Black Death: The Impact of the Fourteenth-century Plague*, Papers of the 11th Annual Conference of the Center for Medieval and Early Renaissance Studies, Medieval and Renaissance Texts and Studies 13, 23–38

Benedictow, O.J., 2004: *The Black Death 1346–53: A Complete History* (Rochester)

Benham, W.G., 1907: *The Oath Book, or Red Parchment Book of Colchester* (Colchester)

Beveridge, W., 1955: 'Westminster Wages in the Manorial Era', *Economic History Review*, ns 8 (1), 18–35

Blackmore, L. and Pearce, J., 2010: *A Dated Type Series of London Medieval Pottery 5: Shelly-sandy ware and the greyware industries* (MoLA Monograph 49)

Blatherwick, S. and Bluer, R., 2004: *Great Houses, Moats and Mills on the South Bank of the Thames* (MoLA Monograph 47)

Boldrick, S., 1997: *The Rise of Chantry Space in England from ca. 1260 to ca. 1400* (PhD Department of Art History and Archaeology, University of Manchester)

Bolton, J., 1996: 'The World Turned Upside Down: plague as an agent of economic and social change', in Ormrod, W.M. and Lindley, P.G. (eds), 1996: *The Black Death in England* (Donington), 17–78

Bowsher, D., Dyson, T., Holder, N. and Howell, I., 2007: *The London Guildhall: an archaeological history of a neighbourhood from early medieval to modern times* (MoLAS Monograph 36: 2 parts + CD-ROM)

Bowsky, W.M., 1964: 'The Impact of the Black Death upon Sienese Government and Society', *Speculum*, 39 (1), 1–34

Braid, R., in prep., *Laying the Foundations for Royal Policy: Economic regulation and market control in London before the Black Death*

Bridbury, A.R., 1973: 'The Black Death', *Economic History Review*, 26, 577–92

Britnell, R.H., 1994: *The Black Death in English Towns*, Urban History, 21 (2), 196–210

——, nd: Colchester Deeds of the Fourteenth and Fifteenth Centuries, from the archives of the Mercers' Company of London, cartulary of Dean John Colet (www.dur.ac.uk/r.h.britnell/Colchester%20Deeds%201.htm, accessed May 2009)

Carlin, M., 1996: *Medieval Southwark* (London and Rio Grande)

Chanter, J.F., 1910: 'Court Rolls of the Manor of Curry Rivel in the Year of the Black Death', *Somerset Archaeological and Natural History*, 46, 85–135

Cloak, J., 2001: *Cottages and Common Fields of Richmond and Kew* (Chichester)

Cohn, S.K., Jr, 2000: 'The Place of the Dead in Flanders and Tuscany: towards a comparative history of the Black Death', in Gordon, B. and Marshall P. (eds), *The Place of the Dead*, 17–43

——, 2002: 'The Black Death: end of a paradigm', *American Historical Review*, 107 (3), 703–38

——, 2003: *The Black Death Transformed: Disease and Culture in Early Renaissance Europe* (London, pb edn)

Courtenay, W.J., 1980: 'The Effect of the Black Death on English Higher Education', *Speculum*, 55 (4), 696–714

Davis, D.E., 1986: 'The Scarcity of Rats and the Black Death: an ecological history', *Journal of Interdisciplinary History*, 16 (3), 455–70

Davis, M., 2010: *London Women and the Economy Before and After the Black Death*, ESRC End of Award Report, RES-000-22-3343. Swindon: ESRC, 2–5

Davis, R.A., 1989: 'The Effect of the Black Death on the Parish Priests of the Medieval Diocese of Coventry and Lichfield', *Bulletin of the Institute of Historical Research*, 62, 85–90

Davis, V., 1993: 'Medieval English Ordination Lists – a London case study', *Local Population Studies*, 50, 51–60

Dewitte, S.N., 2007: *The Paleodemography of the Black Death, 1347–1351: A Thesis in Anthropology* (PhD Pennsylvania State University)

——, 2009: 'The Effect of Sex on Risk of Mortality During the Black Death in London, AD 1349–1350', *American Journal of Physical Anthropology*, 139 (2), 222–34

DeWitte, S.N. and Woods, J.W., 2008: 'Selectivity of Black Death Mortality with Respect to Pre-existing Health', *Proceedings of the National Academy of Sciences USA*, 105 (5), 1436–41

Divers, D., Mayo, C., Cohen, N. and Jarrett, C., 2009: *A New Millennium at Southwark Cathedral: investigations into the first 2000 years*, PCA Monograph 8, 67

Dohar, W.J., 1995: *Black Death and Pastoral Leadership: The Diocese of Hereford in the Fourteenth Century*

——, 2000: 'Since the Pestilence Time: pastoral care in the later middle ages', in Evans, G.R. (ed.), *A History of Pastoral Care*, 169–200

Drancourt, M., Aboudharam, G., Signoli, M., Dutour, O. and Raoult, D., 1998: 'Detection of 400-year-old Yersinia pestis DNA in human dental pulp: an approach to the diagnosis of ancient septicemia', *Proceedings of the National Academy of Sciences USA*, 95, 12637–40

Drancourt, M., Signoli, M., Dang, L.V., Bizot, B., Roux,V.,Tzortzis, S. and Raoult, D., 2007: '*Yersinia pestis Orientalis* in remains of ancient plague patients', *Emerging Infectious Diseases Journal*, 13 (2), February 2007, 332–3

Duffy, E., 1992: *The Stripping of the Altars:Traditional Religion in England, 1400–1580* (Yale)

Duncan, L.L., nd: *Kent Wills of the Prerogative Court of Canterbury* www.kentarchaeology.org.uk/Research/Libr/Wills/WillsIntro.htm (accessed May 2007)

Duncan, C.J. and Scott, S., 2005: 'What Caused the Black Death?', *Postgraduate Medical Journal*, 81, 315–20

Dunn, P., 2003: *After the Black Death: Society and economy in late fourteenth-century Norwich* (PhD University of East Anglia)

Dyer, C., 1980: *Lords and Peasants in a Changing Society: the estates of the Bishopric of Worcester 680–1540* (Cambridge)

Ecclestone, M., 1999: 'Mortality of Rural Landless Men before the Black Death: the *Glastonbury head-tax* lists', *Local Population Studies*, 63, 6–29

Eisen, R.J., Bearden, S.W.,Wilder, A.P., Montenieri, J.A.,Antolin, M.A. and Gage, K.L., 2006: 'Early-phase transmission of *Yersinia pestis* by unblocked fleas as a mechanism explaining rapidly spreading plague epizootics', *Proceedings of the National Academy of Sciences USA*, 103, 15380–5

Ell, S.R., 1979: 'Some Evidence for Interhuman Transmission of Medieval Plague', *Reviews of Infectious Diseases*, 1 (3), 563–6

——, 1985: 'Iron in Two Seventeenth-century Plague Epidemics', *Journal of Interdisciplinary History*, 15, no 3, 445–57

Emery, R., 1967: 'The Black Death of 1348 in Perpignan', *Speculum*, 42 (4), 611–23

Evans, D.H. (ed.), in prep., *Excavations at the Austin Friary, Hull, 1994–9*, East Riding Archaeology

Fenwick, C.C., 2001: *The Poll Taxes of 1377, 1379 and 1381 (3 pts) Records of Social and Economic History*, ns 29 (Oxford, New York)

Fitch, M., 1979: *Testamentary Records in the Archdeaconry Court of London, Vol. 1: 1363–1649*, British Record Society (London)

Fletcher, J.M.J., 1922: 'The Black Death in Dorset 1348–9', *Proceedings of the Dorset Natural History and Antiquarian Society*, 43, 1–14

Fowler, J.T., 1898/99: *Extracts from the Account Rolls of the Abbey of Durham* (Surtees Society,Vol. 99/100)

Gairdner, J. (ed.), 1876: *Gregory's Chronicle: the historical collections of a citizen of London in the fifteenth century* (Camden Society)

Galbraith,V.H. (ed.), 1927: *Anominalle Chronicle 1333–1381* (Manchester)

Galloway, J.A., 2000: 'One Market or Many? London and the grain trade of England', in Trade, *Urban Hinterlands and Market Integration c. 1300–1600*, ed. J.A. Galloway (CMH Working Papers Series No 3, IHR, 2000), 23–43

Gask, G.E., 1926: 'The Medical Staff of King Edward the Third', *Proceedings of the Royal Society of Medicine*, 19 (Section on History of Medicine, 1–16)

Gasquet, F.A., 1893: *The Great Pestilence AD 1348 to 1349: Now commonly known as the Black Death* (London)

Gilchrist, R., 2008: 'Magic for the Dead?', *Journal of the Society for Medieval Archaeology*, 52, 119–60

Gilchrist, R. and Sloane, B., 2005: *Requiem: the medieval monastic cemetery in Britain* (London)

Giles, J.A., 1845: *Chronicon Angliae Petriburgense* (London)

—— (ed.), 1847: *Galfridi le Baker de Swinebroke, Chronicon Angliae temporibus Edwardi II et Edwardi III* (London)

Given-Wilson, C., 2004: *Chronicles: the writing of history in medieval England* (New York and London)

Grimes, W.F., 1968: *The Excavation of Roman and Medieval London* (London)

Goldberg, P.J.P., 1990: 'Urban Identity and the Poll Taxes of 1377, 1379 and 1381', *Economic History Review*, ns 43 (2), 194–216

Gooder, A., 1998: 'Coventry at the time of the Black Death', *Coventry and County Heritage,* No 23.

Gottfried, R.S., 1980: 'Bury St Edmunds and the Populations of Late Medieval English Towns', 1270–1530, *Journal of British Studies*, 20, 1–31

——, 1983: *The Black Death: natural and human disaster in medieval Europe* (London)

——, 1986: Review of Twigg 1985, *Speculum*, 61, 217–9

Grainger, I., Hawkins, D., Cowal, L. and Mikulski, R., 2008: *The Black Death Cemetery, East Smithfield, London* (MoLAS Monograph 43)

Grainger, I. and Phillpotts, C., 2011: *The Cistercian Abbey of St Mary Graces, East Smithfield, London* (MoLA Monograph 44)

Gransden, A., 1957: 'A Fourteenth-Century Chronicle from the Grey Friars at Lynn', *English Historical Review*, 72, 270–8

Haddock, D. and Kieslin, L., 2002: 'The Black Death and Property Rights', *Journal of Legal Studies*, 31, 545–87

Haensch, S., Bianucci, R., Signoli, M., Rajerison, M., Schultz, M., Kacki, S., Vermunt, M., Weston, D.A., Hurst, D., Achtman, M., Carniel, E. and Bramanti, B., 2010: 'Distinct Clones of Yersinia pestis caused the Black Death', *Public Library of Science: Pathogens*, 6 (10), (accessed at www.plospathogens.org/article/info%3Adoi%2F10.1371%2Fjournal.ppat.1001134)

Hallam, H.E., 1984: 'The Climate of Eastern England 1250–1350', *Agricultural History Review*, 32, 124–32

Hamilton-Thompson, A., 1911: 'The Registers of John Gynewell, Bishop of Lincoln for the years 1347–50', *Archaeology Journal*, 68, 301–60

——, 1914: 'The Pestilences of the Fourteenth Century in the Diocese of York', *Archaeology Journal*, 71, 96–154

Hanawalt, B.A., 1993: *Growing Up in Medieval London: The Experience of Childhood in History* (Oxford and New York)

——, 2007: *The Wealth of Wives: Women, law and economy in late medieval London* (Oxford and New York)

Hardy, T.D., 1869–85: *Syllabus of the documents relating to England and other kingdoms contained in the collection known as 'Rymer's Foedera'* (3 vols) (London)

Harding, V., 1992: 'Burial Choice and Burial Location in Later Medieval London', in Bassett, S. (ed.), *Death in Towns: urban responses to the dying and the dead 100–1600* (London and New York), 119–35

Harvey, B.F., 1993: *Living and Dying in Medieval England 1100–1540* (Oxford)

——, 2000: 'Before and After the Black Death: a monastic infirmary in fourteenth-century England', in Ridyard, S.J., *Death, Sickness and Health in Medieval Society and Culture* (Sewanee Mediaeval Studies, 10), 5–31

Harvey, B.F. and Oeppen, J., 2001: 'Patterns of Morbidity in Late Medieval England: A Sample from Westminster Abbey', *Economic History Review*, ns 54 (2), 215–39

Harvey, J.H., 1947: 'Some London Painters of the 14th and 15th Centuries', *Burlington Magazine for Connoisseurs*, 89 (536), 303–5

Hatcher, J., 1986: 'Mortality in the Fifteenth Century: some new evidence', *Economic History Review*, ns 39 (1), 19–38

——, 1994: 'England in the Aftermath of the Black Death', *Past and Present*, 144, 3–35

Hawkins, D., 1990: 'The Black Death and the New London Cemeteries of 1348', *Antiquity*, 64, 637–42

Haydon, F.S. (ed.), 1863: *Eulogium historiarum sive temporis: chronicon ab orbe condito usque as annum domini M.CCC.LXVI*, Vol. 3, Rolls Series (London)

Henderson, J., 1988: 'The Parish and the Poor in Florence at the Time of the Black Death: the case of S. Frediano', in Henderson, J. (ed.), *Charity and the Poor in Medieval and Renaissance Europe, Continuity and Change*, 3 (2), 247–72

Hennessey, G., 1898: *Novum Repertorium Ecclesiasticum Parochiale Londinense: Or, London Diocesan Clergy Succession from the Earliest Time to the Year 1898, with Copious Notes* (London)

Hill, F., 1948: *Medieval Lincoln* (Cambridge)

Hockey, S.F. (ed.), 1986: *The Register of William Edington Bishop of Winchester 1346–1366* (Hampshire Record Series 7) Pt 1

—— (ed.), 1987: *The Register of William Edington Bishop of Winchester 1346–1366* (Hampshire Record Series 7) Pt 2

Hodgett, G.A.J., 1971: *The Cartulary of Holy Trinity, Aldgate* (London)

Hollingsworth, M.F. and Hollingsworth, T.H., 1971: 'Plague mortality rates by age and sex in the parish of St Botolph's without Bishopsgate, London, 1603', *Population Studies*, 25 (1), 131–46

Holt, R.A., 1987: *Gloucester: an English provincial town during the later Middle Ages* (PhD School of History, Faculty of Arts, University of Birmingham)

Horrox, R., 1994: *The Black Death* (Manchester)

——, 2006: Review of Benedictow 2004, *English Historical Review*, 121, 197–9

Hovland, S.R., 2006: *Apprenticeship in Later Medieval London (c. 1300–c. 1530)* (PhD Royal Holloway, University of London)

Hurston, Rev. E., 1856: 'notes', *Proceedings of the Archaeological Institute*, 13, 185–6

Johnson, C. (ed.), 1946–8: *Diocesis Roffensis Registrum Hamonis Hethe*, 2 vols, Canterbury & York Society, 48–9

Jones, B. (ed.), 1964: *Fasti Ecclesiae Anglicanae, 1300–1541, by John Le Neve*, Vol. 10, Coventry and Lichfield Diocese (London)

Jones, R.T., Sly, J., Simpson, J., Rackham, J. and Locker, A., 1985: 'Animal Bones: Report', reproduced in Austin, D., 2007: *Acts of Perception: A study of Barnard Castle in Teesdale* (2 vols), Vol. 2, 589–606

Karlsson, G., 1996: 'Plague without Rats: the case of fifteenth-century Iceland', *Journal of Medieval History*, 22 (3), 263–84

Keene, D., 1984: 'A New Study of London before the Great Fire', *Urban History Yearbook 1984*, 11–21 (Leicester)

——, 1990: 'Shops and Shopping in Medieval London', in Grant, L. (ed.), *Medieval Art, Architecture and Archaeology in London*, British Archaeological Association, Conference Transactions, 10, 29–46

Kingsford, C.L., 1908: *John Stow: A Survey of London* (London), 2 vols

——, 1915: *The Grey Friars of London* (Aberdeen)

Kreider, A., 1979: *English Chantries: the Road to Dissolution* (Cambridge, Mass.)

Laurent, M-H., 1937: *I necrologi di Siena di San Domenico in Camporegio (Epoca Cateriniana)* (Siena)

Levillain, P. (ed.), 2002: *The Papacy: An encyclopaedia*, Vol. 2 (New York)

Liddle, J., 2007: 'Animal Bone', in Lyon, J., *Within these Walls: Roman and medieval defences north of Newgate at the Merrill Lynch Financial Centre, City of London* (MoLAS Monograph 33), 175–6

Lindley, P., 1996: 'The Black Death and English Art: a debate and some assumptions', in Ormrod and Lindley (eds), *The Black Death in England*, 125–46

Logan, F.D., 1996: *Runaway Religious in Medieval England, c. 1240–1540*, Cambridge Studies in Medieval Life and Thought, 4th Series, no 32

Lomas, R.A., 1989: 'The Black Death in County Durham', *Journal of Medieval History*, 15 (2), 127–40

Luard, H.R. (ed.), 1866: *Annales prioratus de Dunstaplia (AD 1–1297); Annales monasterii de Bermundeseia (AD 1042–1432); Annales Monastici iii* (Rolls Series xxxvi) (London)

Lumby, J.R., 1882: *Polychronicon Ranulphi Higden, monachi cestrensis*, Vol. VIII, Rolls Series (London)

Lütgert, S.A., 2000: 'Victims of the Great Famine and the Black Death?' *Hikuin*, 27, 255–64

Martin, G.H. (ed.), 1996: *Knighton's Chronicle 1337–1396* (Oxford)

McCormick, M., 2003: 'Rats, Communications and Plague: toward an ecological history', *Journal of Interdisciplinary History*, 43, 1–25

McHardy, A.K., 1977: *The Church in London, 1375–92* (London)

Bibliography

Megson, B.E., 1996: 'Life Expectations of the Widows and Orphans of Freemen in London 1375–1399', *Local Population Studies*, 57, 18–29

——, 1998: 'Mortality among London Citizens in the Black Death', *Medieval Prosopography*, 19, 125–33

Miller, P. and Saxby, D., *The Augustinian Priory of St Mary Merton, Surrey: Excavations 1976–90* (MoLAS Monograph 34)

Mortimer, I., 2008: *The Perfect King: The Life of Edward III, Father of the English Nation* (Pimlico edn)

Munro, J., 2004: *Before and After the Black Death: Money, Prices, and Wages in Fourteenth-Century England*, Department of Economics and Institute for Policy Analysis, University of Toronto, Working Paper 24

Naphy, W.G. and Spicer, A., 2004: *Plague: Black Death and Pestilence in Europe*

Nightingale, P., 1995: *A Medieval Mercantile Community: the Grocers' Company and the politics and trade of London, 1000–1485* (New Haven & London)

——, 1996: 'The Growth of London in the Medieval English Economy', in Britnell, R.H. and Hatcher, J., *Progress and Problems in Medieval England: essays in honour of Edward Miller* (Cambridge), 89–106

——, 2005: 'Some New Evidence of Crises and Trends of Mortality in Late Medieval England', *Past and Present*, 187, 33–68

Norris, M., 1991: 'Later Medieval Monumental Brasses: an urban funerary industry and its representation of death', in Bassett, S. (ed.), *Death in Towns*, 184–209

Nutton, V. (ed.), 2008: *Pestilential Complexities: understanding medieval plague*, Medical History Supplement, 27

O'Connor, S.J. (ed.), 1993: *A Calendar of the Cartularies of John Pyel and Adam Fraunceys* (Camden Society, 5th Series, Vol. 2)

Olea, R.A. and Christakos, G., 2005: 'Duration of Urban Mortality for the 14th Century Black Death Epidemic', *Human Biology*, 77 (3), 291–303

Orme, N. and Webster, M., 1995: *The English Hospital 1070–1570* (Yale)

Ormrod, W.M., 1989: 'The Personal Religion of Edward III', *Speculum*, 64 (4), 849–77

——, 1996: 'The Politics of Pestilence', in Ormrod and Lindley (eds), *The Black Death in England*, 147–81

Ormrod, W.M. and Lindley, P.G. (eds), 1996: *The Black Death in England* (Donington)

Palmer, R., 1987: Review of Twigg 1985, *Quarterly Review of Biology*, 62, no 1, 124

Parry, J.H., 1912: *Registrum Johannis de Trillek, episcopi Herefordensis*, Canterbury and York Society, Vol. 8

Phillpotts, C.J., 1999: 'The Metropolitan Palaces of Medieval London', *London Archaeologist*, 9 (2), 47–53

Pipe, A., 2007: 'Animal Bone', in Miller and Saxby, *The Augustinian Priory of St Mary Merton, Surrey: Excavations 1976–90*

Prentice, M.B., Gilbert, T. and Cooper, A., 2004: 'Was the Black Death caused by Yersinia pestis?', *Lancet: Infectious Diseases*, 4, 72

Prescott, E., 1992: *The English Medieval Hospital* (London)

Pugh, R.B., 1968: 'Some Medieval Moneylenders', *Speculum*, 43 (2), 274–89

Putnam, B.H., 1908: 'The Enforcement of the Statutes of Labourers during the First Decade after the Black Death 1349–1359', *Studies in History Economics and Public Law*, Vol. 32 (New York)

——, 1915: 'Maximum Wage-Laws for Priests after the Black Death, 1348–1381', *American Historical Review*, 21 (1), 12–32

Raoult, D., Aboudharam, G., Crubezy, E., Larrouy, G., Ludes, B. and Drancourt, M., 2000: 'Molecular Identification by "Suicide PCR" of *Yersinia pestis* as the agent of Medieval Black Death', *Proceedings of the National Academy of Sciences USA*, 97, 12800–3

Raine, J. (ed.), 1886: 'The Continuation of Thomas Stubbs' *chronica pontificum ecclesiae Eboracensis*', in *Historians of the Church of York*, Vol. 2, Rolls Series 71 (London) 428–33

Rawcliffe, C., 2006: *Leprosy in Medieval England* (Woodbridge)

Redstone, V.B. and Redstone, L.J., 1937: 'The Heyrons of London: a study in the social origins of Geoffrey Chaucer', *Speculum*, 12 (2), 182–95

Rees, W., 1923: 'The Black Death in England and Wales as exhibited in manorial documents', *Proceedings of the Royal Society of Medicine* (Section on History of Medicine), 16, 27–45

Reid, T., 1928: *History of the Parish of Crawfordjohn, Upper ward of Lanarkshire, 1153–1928* (Edinburgh)

Rickert, E., 1952: 'Chaucer at School', *Modern Philology*, 29, 257–74

Riley, H.T., 1861: *Liber Albus: The White Book of the City of London* (London)

——, 1863: *The Chronicles of the Mayors and Sheriffs of London, AD 1188 to 1274; The French Chronicle of London, AD 1259 to 1343* (London)

——, 1868: *Memorials of London and London Life in the 13th, 14th and 15th Centuries* (London)

Röhrkasten, J., 2001: 'Trends of Mortality in Late Medieval London (1348–1400)', *Nottingham Medieval Studies*, 45, 172–209

——, 2004: *The Mendicant Houses of Medieval London 1221–1539*, Vita Regularis, Vol. 21 (Münster)

Rosser, G., 1989: *Medieval Westminster* (Oxford)

Rousseau, M., 2003: *Chantry Foundations and Chantry Chaplains at St Paul's Cathedral, London, c. 1200–1548* (PhD Royal Holloway and Bedford New College, University of London)

Rushton, N., 2002: 'Spatial Aspects of the Almonry Site and the Changing Priorities of Poor Relief at Westminster Abbey c. 1290–1540', *Architectural History*, 45, 66–91

Russell, J., 1948: *British Medieval Population* (Albuquerque)

Sabine, E.L., 1933: 'Butchering in Mediaeval London', *Speculum*, 8 (3), 335–53

St John Hope, W., 1925: *The History of the Charterhouse from its Foundation until the Suppression of the Monastery* (London)

Bibliography

Salter, H.E., 1912: *Coroners Inquests, the Walls of Oxford etc.* (Oxford)

Schofield, J., 1995: *Medieval London Houses* (Yale)

Schofield, J. and Lea, R., 2005: *Holy Trinity Priory, Aldgate* (MoLAS Monograph 24)

Scott, S. and Duncan, C.J., 2001: *Biology of Plagues: Evidence from Historical Populations* (Cambridge)

——, 2004: *Return of the Black Death: the World's Greatest Serial Killer*

Sharpe, R.R., 1885: *Calendar of Letters from the Mayor and Corporation of the City of London 1350–1370* (London)

Shaw, A.T., 2000: *Reading the Liturgy at Westminster Abbey in the Late Middle Ages* (PhD Royal Holloway, University of London)

Shrewsbury, J.D.F., 1970: *A History of Bubonic Plague in the British Isles* (Cambridge)

Siraisi, N.G., 1982: 'Introduction', in Williman, D. (ed.), *The Black Death: The impact of the fourteenth-century plague*, Papers of the 11th Annual Conference of the Centre for Medieval and Early Renaissance Studies, Medieval and Renaissance Texts and Studies 13

Sloane, B. and Malcolm, G., 2004: *Excavations at the Priory of the Hospital of St John of Jerusalem, Clerkenwell* (MoLAS Monograph 20)

Steffensen, J., 1974: *Plague in Iceland*, Nordisk Medicinhistorisk Årsbok, 40–55

Sutton, A.F., 2005: *The Mercery of London: Trade, goods and people 1130–1578* (London)

Tait, J., 1914: *Chronica Iohannis de Reading et anonymi Cantuariensis 1346–67* (Manchester)

Theilmann, J. and Cate, F., 2007: 'A Plague of Plagues: the problem of plague diagnosis in medieval England', *Journal of Interdisciplinary History*, 37 (3), 371–93

Thomas, C., Cowie, R. and Sidell, J., 2006: *The Royal Palace, Abbey and Town of Westminster on Thorney Island: Archaeological excavations (1991–8) for the London Underground Limited Jubilee Line Extension Project* (MoLAS Monograph 22)

Thomas, M., Gilbert, P., Cuccui, P., White, W., Lynnerup, N., Titball, R.W., Cooper, A. and Prentice, M.B., 2004: 'Absence of *Yersinia pestis*-specific DNA in human teeth from five European excavations of putative plague victims', *Microbiology*, 150, 341–54

Thompson, E.M. (ed.), 1889a: *Chronicon Galfridi le Baker de Swynebroke* (Oxford)

—— (ed), 1889b: *Robertus de Avesbury de Gestis Mirabilibus Regis Edwardi Tertii* (Rolls Series)

Thompson, J.A.F., 1965: 'Piety and Charity in Late Medieval London', *Journal of Ecclesiastical History*, 16, 178–95

Thrupp, S., 1996: *The Merchant Class of Medieval London* (Michigan, revised edition, 3rd edn)

Tuchmann, B., 1989: *A Distant Mirror: the calamitous 14th century* (London)

Twigg, G., 1984: *The Black Death: a biological reappraisal* (London)

Twiss, T., 1873: *Monumenta Juridica: the Black Book of the Admirality*, Vol. 2 (London)

Tyler, K., 1998: 'Excavations at the Former Allied Brewery 148–180 St John Street London EC1', *Transactions of the London and Middlesex Archaeological Society*, 49, 107–32

Tytler, P.F., 1845: *A History of Scotland, Vol. II (1346–1424)* (3rd edn, 5 vols, Edinburgh)

Weetman, J.F., 2004: *Testamentary Piety and Charity in London, 1259–1370* (PhD, University of Oxford)

Westlake, H.F., 1923: *Westminster Abbey: The church, convent, cathedral and college of St Peter Westminster, London* (2 Vols)

Wilson, B., 2005: 'Animal Bones and Shells', in Page, P., Atherton, K. and Hardy, A., *Barentin's Manor: excavations of the moated manor at Harding's Field, Chalgrove, Oxfordshire 1976–9*, Oxford Archaeology, 125–53

Wilson, C., Gem, R., Tudor-Craig, P. and Physick, J., 1986: *Westminster Abbey* (London)

Wilkinson, L., 1985: Review of Twigg 1985, *Medical History*, 29, no 3, 326–8

Wood, J.W., Ferrell, R.J. and DeWitte-Avina, S.N., 2003: 'The Temporal Dynamics of the Fourteenth-Century Black Death: New evidence from English ecclesiastical records', *Human Biology*, 75 (4), August 2003, 427–48

Wood, J. and DeWitte-Avina, S., 2003: 'Was the Black Death yersinial plague?', *Lancet: Infectious Diseases*, 3, 327–8

Wood-Legh, K.L., 1932: 'Some Aspects of the History of the Chantries during the Reign of Edward III', *Cambridgeshire History Journal*, 4 (1), 26–50

Wray, S., 2005: Review of Benedictow 2004, *Journal of the History of Medicine*, 60, 514–7

Ziegler, P., 1977: *The Black Death* (Stroud)

INDEX

Other titles published by The History Press

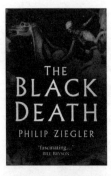

The Black Death
PHILIP ZIEGLER
978-0-7509-3202-8
£13.49

A series of natural disasters in the Orient during the fourteenth century caused the most devastating period of death and destruction in European history. Philip Zeigler's overview of this crucial event synthesises the records of contemporary chroniclers and the work of later historians in one volume. This illustrated narrative presents the full horror and destruction caused by the Black Death.

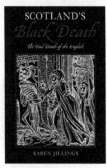

Scotland's Black Death
KAREN JILLINGS
978-0-7524-3732-3
£11.69

During the early months of 1349, Scottish soldiers engaged in border warfare praised God that many of their English opponents were being felled by a new and terrifying affliction. This book describes the social impacts of the plague, such as cynicism towards the Church and the abandonment of serfdom, and demonstrates the way in which they were all integral to the development of the country.

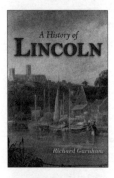

A History of Lincoln
RICHARD GURNHAM
978-1-86077-551-2
£16.19

This fully illustrated book tells the story of Lincoln's many transformations over 2,000 years: as a provincial capital of the Roman Empire; the arrival of the Vikings in the ninth century; as a major centre for the wool and cloth trades in the twelfth and thirteenth centuries; its decline before and after the Black Death struck in 1349; and its rapid growth in the nineteenth century. Through a wealth of detail, the author brings to life the events and challenges faced by many generations who have lived and worked in this city.

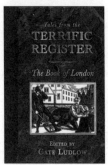

Tales from the Terrific Register: the Book of London
EDITED BY CATE LUDLOW
978-0-7524-5264-7
£8.99

Fast-paced, astonishingly gory and featuring as many corpses as possible, the Terrific Register was a publishing sensation. As a schoolboy, Charles Dickens was never without a copy. This selection contains many tales of London life that will startle the modern reader, including gripping stories of fires, floods and disasters, 'eye-witness' accounts of the great plague and 'the last moment of Lord Balmerino, executed on Tower Hill, 1746'.

Visit our website and discover thousands of other History Press books.

www.thehistorypress.co.uk